The New Black Lace Book
of Women's Sexual Fantasies

The New Black Lace Book of
Women's Sexual Fantasies
Compiled and Edited by Mitzi Szereto

BL

Black Lace books contain sexual fantasies.
In real life, always practise safe sex.

This edition published in 2008 by
Black Lace
Thames Wharf Studios
Rainville Rd
London W6 9HA

Copyright © Virgin Books Ltd and Mitzi Szereto

A catalogue record for this book is available from the British Library.

www.black-lace-books.com

Typeset by Palimpsest Book Production Limited, Grangemouth, Stirlingshire, FK3 8KG

Distributed in the USA by Macmillan, 175 Fifth Avenue, New York, NY 10010, USA

ISBN 978 0 352 34172 3

5 7 9 10 8 6

Penguin Random House is committed to a sustainable future for our business, our readers and our planet. This book is made from Forest Stewardship Council® certified paper.

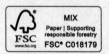

MIX
Paper | Supporting responsible forestry
FSC® C018179

Printed and bound in Great Britain by Clays Ltd, St Ives plc

Contents

Acknowledgements

With thanks to Ashley Lister and Stuart Burrell

'One of the most adventurous things left us is to go to bed. For no one can lay a hand on our dreams.'

— E V Lucas

1

Introduction: Why am I Here and Where are We Now?

Well, I suppose I should explain just how I ended up here in the first place. Perhaps it all goes back to my fifth year in primary school. And no, it's not what you're thinking – no playground rendezvous with the little boys or, for that matter, little girls. Rather my voracious appetite for books and the reading of them led me to borrow from a female classmate a dog-eared copy of the Victorian erotica classic *The Romance of Lust* that belonged to her parents. I became quite engrossed in this smutty tome though, admittedly, some of it went right over my head, which was probably a good thing in retrospect. My downfall came in trying to secrete it inside a school library copy of Abraham Lincoln's biography. My mother thought I seemed just a wee bit too engrossed in the tale of Honest Abe, and consequently I was busted!

I'll admit that my taste in reading material, although it wouldn't be remotely along the same lines as *The Romance of Lust* for a number of years, was strictly adult in nature. Being an extremely precocious child (and an only child at that), I found I couldn't abide the books aimed at my age group; not even the Young Adult novels could capture my fancy. Therefore, I opted to go with either seething Gothic Romances or the potboilers from the bestseller lists. Aside from the fact that the stories were engaging and well-written, there was plenty of sex (or at least a jolly good hint of it) to help a budding young writer of erotic fiction file it away for future inspiration.

As a writer of erotic prose and an editor of it as well, I've worked to expand my brief into the mainstream, crossing into other genres. But the core element of the erotic is always inherent in my work, be it subtle or extreme. As a writer, I consider it my job to create, and this can and does involve fantasy and, occasionally, a bittersweet dose of reality. Sometimes it comes purely (or, for that matter, *impurely*) from the imagination, bearing no relation to personal taste or experience. However, because the erotic is so cerebral, it's not surprising that the writing of it quite often stems from the writer's personal fantasies. Fantasies are our private playground – and you don't need to be a writer to frolic in this sandbox. We're all gifted with the ability to fantasise, and when it comes to sexual fantasy, the scenarios are as varied as the owners of the minds doing the fantasising.

To mark the fifteenth anniversary of Black Lace Books, I am pleased to have been invited to edit this new volume and, indeed, to offer some indication as to where we, as women, are today as sexual beings. The first *Black Lace Book of Women's Sexual Fantasies* is the most successful title in Black Lace's history. Originally published in 1999, it has never been out of print and is still read widely throughout the world. There's a simple reason for this success: the book was authentic. And, indeed, the content of this book is likewise 100 per cent authentic, not solicited scenarios from professional sex writers. While *The New Black Lace Book of Women's Sexual Fantasies* will primarily be upbeat and entertaining, it will also provide an informal sociological and cultural study of contemporary female sexuality in Britain and beyond. Entertainment and enlightenment, surprise and titillation, and, hopefully, some shaking up of assumptions. That is what I'm offering.

As editor, the most important thing for me was to be as representational of the female population as possible. Material has been collected, read and analysed from women of all ages and all sexualities and lifestyles – from women in steady relationships to those who are virgins (and yes, they're out there!), from women who are very sexually active to women who are celibate. I've chosen to include more detailed information for each participant such as age, domestic and sexual lifestyle status, education, profession and location, in order to give a fuller picture of each woman. These are *real* women, not inventions of lad's magazines or the porn industry – real women who have experienced sex and sexual fantasy in a multitude of ways and means. These women have shared their private lives with us and exhibited their secret thoughts to thousands of readers. Their courage and honesty should be applauded. It would be hubris to categorise (and thus draw conclusions from) women's sexual interests and fantasies according to age, education, and profession, and I won't even attempt to do so. As is evident on these pages, women are truly all over the map as far as the content of their fantasies. In fact, it's probably safe to say that it would be a major mistake to assume *anything* about a woman based on age, education or profession.

Since the publication in 1999 of the first *Black Lace Book of Sexual Fantasies*, the sexual landscape has changed dramatically. Sexual habits, lifestyles, opportunities and the possibilities for women have been affected by a whole range of new influences, technologies and media. In many ways 1999 seems a more innocent time than that in which we now find ourselves. Everything has become so complicated – the more choices given to us and the more variety of means in which we have to enjoy them, the more we keep searching and seeking. We now live in a world of internet dating, whether of an adult nature (offering no-strings sex as well as avenues for marrieds looking to play outside the marital home), to providing online access to those with more traditional romantic aspirations. There are sites for swingers and sites for the marriage-minded. There are sites for young women looking for rich sugar daddies and sites for older women looking for younger men. Whichever option one chooses, they have created easy access to numerous partners or potential partners. Now women don't even need to step out of their front door to find a man. The internet has become the proverbial singles' bar, revolutionising sexual and dating habits. No longer is it necessary to rely on friends or work mates to 'fix us up' or, for that matter, to sit at a bar nursing a glass of wine for an entire evening in the hope that a man will take the initiative to start up a conversation. As a result, the popularity of internet dating has led to a surge in female promiscuity.

Surprisingly, for a large number of people, the sites aimed at the relationship-minded seem to have become just the opposite, offering a less stigmatised way for those seeking no-strings sex, thereby eliminating the need to join the 'adult' sites catering for those simply 'on the prowl'. It should, however, be mentioned that these sites have also been covertly used by marrieds claiming to be single, especially in the case of men – meaning don't always believe everything you read on the tin!

The rise of recreational sex (swinging) has also had an impact on women's sexual habits, specifically when it comes to married women or women in steady relationships. Sexual fantasies and the willingness of these women to live them out have led many to discard monogamy as a lifestyle choice. Although statistically the numbers in the swinging community are not high, the openness of participants and the media's prurient spotlight upon it make recreational sex appear more prevalent than it actually is. Nevertheless, it's definitely out there and a lot easier to find for those who wish to find it.

Locating partners to have sex with is one thing, but now it seems there are even more ways in which to actually have sex – how does one choose? In the last decade there has been a proliferation of hardcore pornography in visual media, and a rise and mainstreaming of kink. Sex and porn appear in popular music, advertising, talk shows and reality TV. Without a doubt, pornography has had an influence on contemporary sexual culture, and that hasn't changed. If anything, it's exposed the general population to acts they would never have dreamed of, let alone imagined being physically or physiologically possible. It can also be argued that it's had a desensitising effect, particularly on men. Twenty-first century porn is embellished with alternative sexual practices, and even extreme sexual practices, leading to a rise in what is often dubbed 'Freak-show Porn'. Fisting (originally a practice among the gay leather community) and squirting (the medical verdict is still out on this one) can easily be found in porn, as well as gang-bang scenarios, some of which can be extremely brutal. It's also becoming common to witness double, if not triple, penetration, very often in the same orifice (reconstructive surgeons for porn stars are already having a lucrative field day with the physiological results). Every sexual taste and perversion is catered for and, thanks to the internet and a broadband connection, available at the click of a mouse.

In recent years sex toys have enjoyed a massive increase in popularity, availability and variety. Once objects of embarrassment, they have now become accepted and have made their way into the mainstream, enhancing the sex lives of women who are either with or without partners. No longer is it considered unusual for a woman to have at least one toy in her bedside drawer or, for that matter, to include a stop at her local

Ann Summers as part of her Saturday afternoon shopping. More and more heterosexual couples are discovering the fun of adding sex toys to their bedroom repertoire, thereby improving their sex lives and bringing them closer together.

Today's woman is definitely a lot more open about what she wants in the bedroom – and that's a good thing. And, although the mass media and pornography would like us to believe that women are getting it and getting it good, this is not always the reality. According to the women who have participated in our survey, it's a pretty mixed bag. While some women are having the time of their lives, others are still waiting for *the one* to ring their bell, while others are hoping to recreate that singularly amazing experience that transformed their lives. Therefore, if we are to draw any sort of conclusion from all of this, the sexual experiences and sexual satisfactions of the contemporary woman are *not* the same. Meaning – there *is* no norm, and women should not be made to feel in any way wanting because their sexual experiences do not compare with or measure up to others. Be it the lack of a suitably satisfying partner (or a partner in general), the stress of work and family life, health issues, disability, etc., women are not all the same – and neither are their sex lives. However, one thing that *does* appear to be universal is the modern woman's willingness to try new things, to experiment, to abandon her inhibitions, even if only in her fantasy life. The variety of sexual activity discussed in the questionnaires and explored in the fantasies submitted to this project indicate that women are definitely more open and up for new things in the erotic arena, and can not only compete with, but may even have surpassed their male counterparts in both sexual imagination and experiment- ation. Maybe with a bit of courage and the right partner, all these women will one day be able to live out their fantasies, providing, of course, that they wish to or, at the very least, are able to share their fantasies with those with whom they share their bodies, thereby leading to a richer and more fulfilling sex life.

I'd like to thank the many participants who sent in their questionnaires. They came in from every corner of the world, including Great Britain, Ireland, the United States, Canada, Austria, Germany, Sweden, the Netherlands, Australia, New Zealand, South America, China, Singapore, Korea, Kenya, and even Botswana. Without these women willing to share themselves and their sexual thoughts with us, this book would not have been possible. I was touched by many of the replies, some of which were highly personal and heartfelt about these women's private lives and feelings, their hopes and disappointments. Even with the anonymity provided, it could not have been easy for them to open themselves so completely to both myself and you, the reader.

By the way, one of the fantasies in this book is mine. Can you guess which one?

2

The Simple Pleasures

'Simplicity is the glory of expression.'
 – Walt Whitman

When we fantasise, we embark upon journeys that take us to places we're never likely to visit or experience. This holds particularly true when it comes to the realm of the erotic. Fantasies are our private haven, our safety net, the place where we can imagine anything and everything and be completely free from judgement or censure. We can remove ourselves from our daily humdrum realities. We can become someone else, be as wild as we desire, do things we'd never consider doing, have sex with people we'd never in our lives consider having sex with. There are no limits to what we can do inside our minds.

Yet sometimes we don't have to grasp for the extravagant in order to fulfil our desires. Instead we might fantasise about things that are more known to us, things we might already have experienced in some form or other, or can very easily experience given the right set of circumstances. Sometimes a sexual fantasy can be far closer, far more real, offering us a taste of the probable rather than the improbable. Indeed, these fantasies are no less intense or erotic for their simplicity, but are perhaps all the sweeter for it.

There are many ways to enjoy sex – from the sacred to the profane. However, let's begin by getting our feet wet with more traditional pursuits. In this section we will explore the so-called 'vanilla' pleasures – sex that takes place between two consenting adults and that tends not to go too far into the experimental, although it might tease provocatively at the surface. Romantic settings and scenarios are rife, as are encounters between committed partners or those already known to us in some capacity. Historical backdrops are a proven turn-on in this category, steamy bodice-rippers being alive and well in the minds of our participants. So, too, is sex with strangers or those whom we've never met (or are likely to), including a famous country and western music star. It's all in the name of good, clean (well, maybe not *that* clean) fun! Although these fantasies are more concerned with the light than the dark, they are by no means predictable or mundane. For women's sexuality is anything *but* predictable or mundane.

Two's Company

Nicole, age 26
Bisexual
Celibate
Children
Associate's degree
Student
New York, USA

The best sex I probably ever had was with a girl I'd been in the army with. We were stationed in Iraq together and it was my birthday that night. Most of our friends had stayed over in her room and I didn't intend on anything happening. But when I caught a glimpse of her breasts silhouetted against the moonlight, I felt the stirring growing inside my body, pushing against my nipples and thumping against my clitoris. Little by little all of our friends began to leave and I sat next to her on the bed. As if she could sense what I was thinking, she motioned to one of our friends that she was tired and had to go to sleep. I said that I was going to stay over with her since we had not seen each other for a few months. The minute our friend had left, my hands were against her breasts and our tongues were inside each other's mouths, entangled, licking and sucking each other's lips and mouths, our hands rubbing and massaging each other's breasts and nipples, teasing each other. I began kissing her neck until I couldn't take it anymore; I had to have her tits in my mouth. I lifted her shirt and stared at her white breasts with her hard pink nipples protruding as if pushing against an invisible wall. They looked so juicy to me that I swear I'd begun to salivate as my clit hardened, and I could feel the pulse of my heart thudding inside my pants, my tongue seeming to extend itself on its own, as if becoming its own entity. I felt her shiver in my arms as her left nipple entered my wet mouth. I heard her moan a little but I wasn't done. The idea of us getting caught had turned me on so much that I'd begun to play with myself as I kept sucking her tits. I could feel her nipples become harder in my mouth as I licked and sucked faster and faster. I even took both tits and sucked both nipples at the same time. She howled as I nibbled on them, then licked them back and forth like a windshield wiper. Then she lifted off my shirt and sucked my brown nipples as if they spouted water like a fountain.

As I watched her I wanted to come so hard, and my clit felt as hard as a rock and as large as the top of my thumb. Then she placed her hand down my pants and fingered my pussy. I stopped breathing as her fingers fucked me and my clit throbbed with delight. I told her to bite down on my tits and, when she did, the ecstasy was too much to hold inside. I wanted to eat her, to taste her against my tongue. My pants were off in a matter of seconds and so were the rest of her clothes. Naked, we pressed our bodies into each other, feeling the heat of our skin and throb of our clits. I lay on the bed and spread my legs and she lay on top of me, ass first. I could see her wet pussy aching for my tongue and as I plunged it into her she shook and did the same to me. I could feel her tongue inside my hole, licking and sucking inside me. I moaned; it felt so good. I arched my back so she would fall deeper into me and when she did, I could feel her body eating me with excitement. I was so turned on by then, I let my tongue and teeth nibble gently against her clit until I could feel the heat coming off from the inside of her pussy. I let my tongue slip back inside and swallowed her juices. Then I kissed the outside of her pussy lips, letting them slide up and down my lips and tongue. I let my mouth search her clit a little more as her head bobbed up and down, forcing her tongue into my hole. I could feel it fucking me over and over and I was urged to do one better for her.

I put my two fingers into her pussy and fucked her. She was so turned on that she stopped and moved with my fingers. I saw her hips moving back and forth following the motion of my fingers inside her. Then I swirled them a little and she came. She jumped off me and went to her drawer and grabbed her electric dildo and turned it on. I spread my legs and she pushed it into me and then licked my clit at the same time. I pushed her head deeper between my legs and she motioned the dildo faster and faster. I let go of her head and played with my own nipples. She lifted her head to eye level and watched as my nipples were massaged by my hands. I felt the tremor of coming shoot from deep inside me. As I came, she stuck her tongue in my pussy and licked it up, sucking in my juices as they flowed out of me. I grabbed her head as she lapped up all my come into her mouth. Afterwards she climbed on top of me and we kissed with the taste of each other on our lips.

I usually fantasise several times a day. My favourite fantasy is based on the memory of my first sexual experience. I remember when I was fifteen I had my first sexual experience on a staircase with a boy I met at a mock trial conference. His name was Jason and he seemed so nice. As we kissed that night, I had begun to feel urges I had never felt before. So as he lead me up the staircase I was a little afraid and titillated because my mother's apartment was right below where we were. I felt his strong lips kiss mine and the hardness of his cock in his pants. My nipples had begun to protrude through the shirt I was wearing as he massaged my tits. Then he kissed my nipples inside the shirt and I remember this surge ran through my body. It was the first time I had felt something like that and I went wild. I immediately lifted my shirt and I saw his eyes widen with delight. His tongue was large and long and he began to lick my nipples. I moaned his name over and over, and that's when I pulled his cock out. It was the first time I had seen an actual penis not on TV, so when he stroked it with his hands I saw it flex and stretch. As if by instinct, I bent on my knees and put it in my mouth. He moaned and he pushed my head back and forth. I kept sucking as he begged me not to stop. I felt it harden inside my mouth and I sucked even faster until he came in my mouth. I could feel the warm gush of his come sliding down my throat and it tasted so good to me then. As he guided me up, he kissed my lips and his tongue was back in my mouth. Then he went for my nipples again. I arched my legs up as we dry fucked. Then he put his hands down my pants and stroked my clit and pussy. I moaned his name over and over as I felt the power of his lips and hands until my body jerked and I came for the first time.

Name withheld, age 36
Heterosexual
Celibate
Children
College
Social Worker
Nevada, USA

I'm still discovering my sexuality. I was married for fifteen years and sex was OK. I think my ex tried to please me out of obligation. I've always loved vampire films and, even as a little girl, I got a guilty pleasure out of watching the vampire seduce the woman he wanted the most, finally taking her into his arms and biting her ever so tenderly. I've always liked watching and reading porn, especially when the guy is performing oral sex on the woman. I don't mind watching the woman masturbate, but I look for men masturbating. It's really hard to find. I think of myself as a voyeur because I don't feel at liberty to have intercourse. I knew from a young age that I was straight. Although there was this one time, I don't know how it came about, but I kissed this girl. I was probably eight years old. I liked it OK, but preferred boys by far and never told anyone (I think) until now.

Growing up in a poor black neighbourhood for a few years, sex was not looked upon favourably by my grandmother or mother. Although I was intrigued by sex, I feared doing it because I was afraid of getting pregnant. My mom had me at fourteen and instilled a fear in me that she would find out if I ever did it. I spent a lot of years in church and that influenced me a lot, much to my ex's dismay. There were things that Christian women didn't do, and I liked the idea of doing them all, but was afraid to for some reason. I've relaxed over the years, but now I'm divorced. I have had sex (unfortunately) with a guy that I was very attracted to, but the sex wasn't what I expected. He had stamina, but that's not what I want. I really want intimacy mixed with roughness. I don't know if I like it for sure, because I've never had the opportunity, but I'd love to be tied up. I'd be a risk taker . . . risky for frigid me. What holds me back? God, mostly. I had a guy ask me once (when I was married), if I felt it did not have any negative repercussions, would I do it. I told him no. He asked why. I said because I'd know what I'd done. I don't want to be promiscuous even though I love men and would like to be with them physically. Trade salvation for orgasm? I think I'm doing it anyway, but don't feel that great about it. Sometimes I wish I didn't have a sex drive. It reminds me that I'm human.

The best sex I ever had was when my ex and I were first married. He's in the military and at the time we were stationed in England. His tour was up there, so the house was packed up and we were waiting for our time to leave. We had sex about every other day back then, almost like clockwork. This one particular morning we had sex, but I didn't care for it because it seemed one-sided and I got absolutely nothing out of it. I started crying and he asked me what was wrong. I told him that I didn't think the sex was good. I don't remember if he said anything, but he started touching me (I really can't remember how). I was ready to receive him and he entered me – missionary style. It was slow and deliberate. I could feel the arch in his lower back as he gently thrust his penis in and out of me. I began to move my pelvis when it started feeling good to me. We got in sync with each other. At some point he rubbed me just right. Our pace quickened and I felt the shudder that told me that orgasm was imminent. This caused me to move . . . with more enthusiasm. He was really close to coming but didn't climax. Then I felt it, that inexplicable rush that only seems to come with intercourse climaxes. I convulsed (I can't think of another way to put it) and held him close as he continued his motions. Then he came and we were on the floor in the living room coming together. That was a good day.

The main theme running through my fantasies is that the man really wants to be with me and it's not about the sex, but the intimacy of two people joining together in the most physical way possible. He holds me tightly and seems to never want to let me go. In my favourite fantasies a guy who's a friend has recently caused me to have two massive orgasms without ever penetrating my vagina with his penis. These fantasies, if they can be called that, are basically him teaching me what he knows about oral sex and different forms of foreplay. He ties me up. He bathes me and then licks me. He buys me leather and I wear it for him so he can playfully torment me until I beg for his mouth to eat me.

Rachael, age 21
Heterosexual
Single, moderately sexually active
National Vocational Qualification
Store Assistant
East Midlands, UK

I fantasise about women, although I have had no sexual experiences with any. I fantasise about lots of men taking advantage of me and being watched as I masturbate. I love erotic books; I also enjoy porn movies (especially girl on girl). I enjoy sending people video messages of myself masturbating and finding out they're horny and want their cocks deep inside me!

In my favourite fantasy I'm a passenger in a car with a friend (male). We haven't planned anywhere to go or anything to do. As we drive, a storm begins. I tell him storms turn me on and before I know it I'm playing with my clit in the passenger seat. He pulls over in a quiet country lane, and I can see his trousers bulging. He rips open my shirt and gropes my breasts. I become increasingly turned on as he fumbles to find his way inside my trousers. When he touches me I scream with pleasure and orgasm so fast that, before I know it, we're on the back seat of the car, my legs spread so wide as he thrusts deep into me.

Jeanne, age 81
Heterosexual
Widowed, celibate but looking
Children
Author/Pensioner
Wiltshire, UK

I fell madly in love with Errol Flynn at ten years old, though I knew nothing about sex then. In film I was also turned on by *The Three Musketeers* and *Dracula*, particularly the bit where Jonathan Harker is seduced by Dracula's vampire bride/sisters. I loved the hippy era, where men wore flowing hair and kaftans, loons and sandals, and lots of beads. I've always been a bohemian in dress and taste. Then there were the dashing cavaliers of the seventeenth century, again long hair and fancy clothes, with much swashbuckling and swordplay. This was down to early reading of historical novels. Turn-ons now are Johnny Depp in *The Libertine* and male ballet dancers in classical and modern pieces.

My fantasies feature young handsome men with long hair and chiselled features. I'm cynical now, no longer romantic, but I'd still like to find a knight on a white horse to carry me away to Neverland. I like young men, and this is difficult to fulfil now that I'm older. In my fantasy I'm in a pub in Glastonbury. This ancient town is one of my favourite stomping grounds, absolutely heaving with personable young men, the long-haired hippy type that turns me on. I'm at the bar, ordering a G&T. A guy comes in, a Cap'n Jack Sparrow look-alike. I have noticed that several are aping *The Pirates of the Caribbean*. This one in particular has tight jeans, a promising bulge, a baggy-sleeved white shirt, gold hoop earrings, locks halfway down his back and a headscarf.

I want him.

'That one's mine,' I warn off Maggie, the friend I came in with. She nods and shrugs. I know he isn't her bag. She's into the sophisticated male, but is happy to indulge me. Following her own agenda, she heads off in the direction of half a dozen business executives who are slumming it.

I feast my eyes on my boy. It doesn't matter that I'm twice his age. I have always gone for men who are my juniors. Don't find those of my own years in the least attractive. They don't rouse my lust, stir my blood, or fill me with the desire to stroke their curls or unzip their pants. I lean on the bar, eyeing him boldly, never mind that he may think I'm his mother. So what? Isn't there such a thing as an Oedipus complex? I'd spoil him, indulge him, buy him whatever he wanted. I'm not proud.

I've kept my looks, worked on my figure, dress trendy, not frumpy.

'Come to me, baby,' I croon inwardly. 'Let me hire a room, take you upstairs and give you the benefit of my considerable experience and the best blow job of your entire life.'

He drops his money and bends to retrieve it. So do I. Our

fingers meet. I don't draw back and neither does he. He grins and there's that flash of chemistry between us without which sex rarely, if ever, happens. I'm creaming my panties for him. I smile across at Maggie. She shrugs and takes herself off in pursuit of her own ovarian stimulation, knowing what I'm like and leaving me to it. She's on the hunt, following a quest of her own.

'Can I buy you a drink?' is my opening gambit.

'Sure,' he says, glancing at the mates who are with him, some dressed as pirates, too. They give him the thumbs up.

I don't intend to get him plastered – just enough alcohol to make him unaware of the age gap. This doesn't seem to be bothering him, however, and we sit together on a bench. We don't talk much, maybe remark on the historic building, and he tells me he's in a band (what else?), plays guitar and they are going on tour soon. I could be talking to my youngest son. I don't care about this. All I want is to be alone with him. I lean closer, my thigh pressed to his, feeling his heat through my thin skirt. Thrills run up and down my spine and my cunt spasms. It has been some time since I've had one who so closely fulfils my ideal. He's lovely, and I shall be sorry to see him leave.

'Shall we go outside?' he murmurs, his stubbly jaw brushing my cheek. He even smells nice, of joss sticks and patchouli oil and the faint whiff of cannabis.

'Better than that,' I promise, and leave him for a moment to visit the reception desk. It's all so easy if you have money.

We go along the main corridor and mount the curving oak staircase. I have the key for Room 14, the gateway to paradise.

It is everything I had requested of the receptionist, darkly panelled and with a log fire burning in the stone grate. (Mock electric but no matter.) There are velvet drapes at the windows and the pièce de résistance is the massive four-poster bed.

'Cool,' remarks my pick-up, Luke.

'Come on, then, pirate! Show me how you rape and pillage!' I urge, already sprawling over the duvet.

It amuses me to see that he is rather shy, but this is endearing. Does his mummy know he's out? I spend a second speculating on his background. Is he really a drop-out or is this simply a pose? Maybe a student? Does it matter? No. He joins me on the bed, carrying the bottle of wine and two glasses. We drink. Then I've had enough of fucking about and want to get down to business. I take off his bandanna and his long black hair comes snaking down, making him even more irresistible. God, but he's a handsome beast!

He's swarthy, with dark eyes, sort of Italian looking. I push open his shirt and his skin is tanned. His chest carries a sprinkling of hair that thins out, like an arrow pointing past his navel to be swallowed up in the inky thatch covering his lower belly. Losing any reserve he might have had, he holds me in his arms and kisses me. His kisses are thorough, lips, tongue, teeth, everything. Moist and warm and fragrant. Not a hint of halitosis.

I want to screw, yet want it to last. I remind myself that he is young, so could probably perform several times in a row, unlike older men who have to rest after they've shot their bolt. Even so, 'Slow down,' I say, and tug at his belt.

The mattress sags as he sits on one side and pulls off his trainers. White socks follow and then he stands up, wearing only his jeans. He unzips and peels them off, presenting his tight buttocks to me, then turning so that I can see the complete emergence of his cock. What a beauty! It is all that I had hoped for and more, long, already at full stand, brown-skinned and *au naturel*. No knife had robbed him of his foreskin.

'Are you going to let me fuck you?' he asks, with a boyish grin.

'Try and stop me!' I growl, and grab him in a bear-hug. Common sense prevails and I get a packet from my bag, rip it open and take out a silvery condom.

He stands before me and I revel in the pleasurable task of preparing his rock-hard dick. I lick it from base to tip, concentrating on the flange, feeling him shudder, hearing him moan, slurping the milky tears that emerge from the slit. He is oh-so ready. I take care not to tip him over the edge and lose that first, fierce rush of spunk. I slip the rubber on from tip to base. I wish I didn't have to cover that delicious cock but needs must.

I keep him on the boil, working my tongue around his peat-dark nipples, closing on the taut nubs, making him gasp. He takes control, pushing me on my back, parting my legs and going down on me, his face buried in my wet minge. He holds my labial wings apart and sucks my clit, drawing it between his lips. I want to come so badly. He slurps and licks, his tongue-tip giving me divine sensations. My climax breaks and I yell, bucking on the bed, fireworks exploding in my brain. Then he's on me and in me, my knees pressed apart, his cock entering easily despite its size, lubricated by my love-juice.

It's wonderful and he rides me fiercely, coming in savage thrusts. I feel his heat filling the condom. He jerks once, twice, thrice, and then rests his head on my shoulder, breathing quickly and muttering, 'That was wicked! You're one hell of a fuck!'

If I was a cat, I'd purr. What a compliment! My kids would never believe it. And what about my husband who tells me I'm too middle-aged and that no one else but him would be interested in me? I know he's banging his young secretary. Screw you! I think savagely.

I'm far from finished with lover-boy, just warming up. 'On your back,' I command.

I sit astride him, knees on each side of his body, then go higher until I'm straddling his face. He gobbles at my cunt eagerly, his tongue swirling around my engorged clit. I grab him by that lovely hair, using it as a rein to bind him to me. I let myself go, another orgasm rising in waves, taking me to heaven again. I peak, yelling, digging my nails into his scalp. Then, leaving his mouth, I slither down, impaling myself on his upwards-pointing prick.

I take it deep inside me, pumping hard, determined to bring him off. He flips me over, wanting to be on top, and I clamp my legs around his waist as he rams harder, releasing a further hot spurt of come into the condom. It is time we changed this. I don't want a little accident, although I could always say it was my husband's. Neither do I want to pick up something nasty with a long name and fatal results.

We lie there satiated for the moment. The condom is replaced by another.

'You want some more?' He seems surprised and impressed.

'Am I too much for you?'

'Hell, no!' he protests, his manhood under question.

He is utterly charming and I'll have to keep a tight hold on my emotions. Don't want to turn into a pathetic older woman who is besotted with her toyboy.

We drink more wine, and he is obviously intrigued by his surroundings. 'I'm used to sleeping on people's floors or in tents. Never seen anything like this. Only in movies. It must have cost.'

Is he getting mercenary? The thought pops into my mind. I hope not, though it's hard to kid myself that he's there for the sake of my girlish figure and lovely face. I'm not that dumb. He's dipped his wick twice, and the first urgency will be gone. Good thing I lit the candles. It's always more flattering.

I change the subject. 'Have you ever had a massage?'

'One of the girls on a stall at the pop festival was doing them. It was cool.'

Bitch! How dare she touch his body? I'm jealous and determined to put this right.

'Roll over,' I command.

I oil my hands, admiring him all the while. There is something so appealing about a young man's body. His arms are folded and his face rests on them, turned to one side. His shoulders are wide and ripple with muscle. His torso sweeps down to a narrow waist. His buttocks are tight, more muscle-moulding plains and hollows, and his thighs meld into the backs of his knees, his calves, ankles, and tapering feet. I could watch him for ever.

I start at the nape of his neck after pushing aside those raven curls. He lies still as if sleeping, perfectly relaxed. I've learned how to give a massage and, almost gloating, allow my worshipping hands to knead his flesh. I know he is enjoying the sensation, though he doesn't stir. Along his spine, working the sinews like dough, absorbing his youth, masculinity and sexuality through my fingers, then around his supple waist, enjoying the curve of his lower back, diving between his arse cheeks, so excited that I can hardly function.

I get a grip, promise myself a treat very soon, and continue to work on his thighs, knees, lower leg, and finish with his Achilles heel, thinking of Brad Pitt in the movie *Troy*. Luke could be a film star. I daydream of introducing him to a director I know, wondering if he could act. But then, if he were successful, I'd have to share him with a million cock-struck fans. I decide not.

He stirs a little restlessly and I guess that his prick is getting excited again under my ministrations. I'm glad I've another packet of three. I work around each toe.

'D'you want me to turn over?' he murmurs.

'Oh, yes,' I reply, straightening up as he moves with the grace of an athlete, presenting me with the wonderful sight of his dick.

I was right. It's swollen to half mast again.

I give myself a stern talking-to. Don't go for it right away. Concentrate on the rest of him. Leave his bits till last. I obey, and there's tingling anticipation in deliberately avoiding his intimate parts. But he is unable to hide anything from me and, before long, his penis is stiff, pointing upwards like a flagpole. He is unable to control his urges as he attempts to bring this mighty weapon within range of my busy hands. I get a kick out of tormenting him. So near and yet so far. Skimming around the base of his cock, tickling his balls, circling his navel, tweaking his puckered nipples, then bending and dropping a kiss on the mushroom-shaped dickhead. It is red and weeping needy tears.

'Do me!' he begs at last.

I've been waiting for this, testing myself to the limit, determined not to weaken until he asks.

'You really want me to?' I whisper, my cunt hurting with longing, my clit throbbing.

'Bloody hell!' He grabs one of my hands and plonks it on his knob.

This is too much. I'm kneeling on the floor while he mounts me, doggy-fashion. I'm rubbing my clit and coming. He pumps like crazy, throwing back his head and barking. His sperm bursts hotly into the rubber. I fall flat on the carpet with him on top of me. I rejoice in being squashed by this rampant male, a thing of little consequence before the power of his passion. Jeez! This isn't like me! Am I getting soft or something?

He lifts me and he is tender. We're under the covers, his arm around me, my head pillowed on his chest. Our pulses are slowing and we are so comfortable together. 'Can I see you again?' he wants to know.

I have been rather dreading this question. It would be terribly easy for me to fall in love with him and I don't want to be hurt. 'Why? Because I'm a good fuck?' I ask, not really wanting to know.

'Because you are a lovely lady.' He is sincere – for the moment.

'We'll see,' I prevaricate, thinking, it was great while it lasted, and I'll make it last that little bit longer. 'I've booked the room for the night.'

When I'm lonely now and wanting to feed a sexual fantasy I remember this.

Reader, I married him!

We were together 25 years until he died in 2002.

T, age 47
Bisexual
Single, occasionally sexually active
High School diploma
State worker
Massachusetts, USA

It takes a man to know what he's doing to get me to peak to orgasm as opposed to when I was younger, when all it took was a touch. I prefer passion versus just jumping into sex right away. I like to be kissed and touched and hugged. My favourite position is on top with a good hard strong penis. I like to ride. What holds me back is not being able to find a man who feels the same way. They all seem to be selfish and quick, or they just don't know how. The one or two that knew how are already taken (married). That's a turn-off after a while. What turns me on is being with an attractive female, making love to her the way I want to be made love to. Also feeling the hard body of

24

a good-looking man moving all over me and letting me ride him to orgasm. I do wish I knew how to approach females (I'm in the closet). I don't know how to go about finding females that are bi or gay. I'd very much like to explore that avenue now. I've only been with a woman twice in my life and I very much enjoyed it. I find myself looking at attractive females. I fantasise about what it would be like to have sex with them and what I'd like to do to them – how I'd hold them or kiss them and where, how I'd like to bring them to orgasm.

Naja, age 37
Heterosexual
Celibate
No children
Some college
Customer Service Representative
Michigan, USA

I like men who are self-confident, but not condescending. A confident man tends to be a great lover. I have always loved books and words. I love to have a man talk/whisper in my ear or neck. I fantasise several times a day. Since I am in a current dry spell, my fantasy is an oldie but goodie. I would just like to have my brains screwed out. Very little talking or politeness is involved. Just fucking.

Karen, age 33
Heterosexual
Live-in relationship/marriage
Children
Health Advisor/University student
Southeast England, UK

Sexy men turn me on. For me, sexy is a brilliant mind, dry wit, relaxed and easygoing, beautiful expressive eyes, a toned body, long fingers, a smile, etc., etc. No one man has to possess all these qualities, one or more will do. What is sexy about the above list is the person behind them – basically a man who's mysterious, mischievous and self-confident.

In my earlier years my sexual imagination was based purely on how a man looked – i.e., he must be good-looking. Now I want to look beyond what I see. My sexual imagination is sparked by curiosity. I can now look at a man on the train with a frazzled expression over his laptop and think, 'I wonder how he looks in the throes of passion or when he's just come?' I then want to dig deeper to find out what makes him laugh out loud. A few moments later I've created a complete fantasy, ending with him sliding a hand up my skirt and a quick hot fuck in the (train) toilets. Interesting to note that, early on, the men in my fantasies all looked the same – that is, they were black men with big dicks. That's pretty much how it was in reality, so I limited myself. Now I go there mentally with any man with an average dick, because now it's more about the sexual tension between the characters, how he uses his dick and the foreplay involved.

My favourite fantasy is a late evening encounter at the gym in an empty studio with my personal trainer. I've not put it into words before, but will attempt to do so now. I'd never met James this late before for training. I usually saw him in the mornings, but he called early to cancel our morning session and rescheduled it for 9 p.m. 'Car problems,' he'd said. As soon as I arrived we began our workout – none of our usual chit-chat and easy banter I noticed, and he pushed me harder than he'd ever done before. I'd had a stressful day myself so I welcomed the challenge.

I felt the tension draining from my body as we began sparring.

I quite liked this part of the workout because I pretended James was the source of my frustration, and I kicked and punched at him with force. As the workout got more intense, our eyes locked and we began communicating silently. His eyes challenged me to work harder and vent, and mine told him that I would. 'Why are you so frustrated?' hazel eyes asked. 'Because I'm horny and I really, really want to fuck you!' brown eyes responded. 'Really!' his eyes narrowed and mine narrowed in return. We retraced our steps until I was backed against the wall. Without taking his eyes off mine, he slid off his protective hand gear and I slid off my gloves. I took a drink and he took off the protective leg gear I was kicking against. All this time our eyes never strayed from each other's. He walked towards me and held out his hands. I slipped mine into his and he pulled me close. My breathing became erratic and almost stopped when his lips touched mine. It was so gentle my eyes closed and my legs felt weightless. James backed me against the wall and slipped open my mouth with his tongue. He tasted of sex and that raised my pulses to a new level. I sucked gently on his lower lip while he teased my top lip. His hands delivered little electric shocks wherever they went. He groped my ass and pulled me hard towards him so that I could feel his rigid erection. I began to moan quite loudly, which echoed around the empty studio. I opened my eyes when his hands slipped into my leotard and found my wet pussy. 'Can I touch you?' his eyes asked. 'Hell yes!' mine responded. He slipped his finger inside my wetness and I groaned deeply. I began to grind against his finger and slipped my hand inside his shorts. As I touched him I felt my body go weak against him and the kiss deepened. His cock was hot and throbbing, hard as steel. I could hear our pleasure sounds reverberating around the empty room. I longed for him to lay me down and bury his cock inside me. The only light in the room was the slits of street lighting through the blinds so I couldn't see him very well. I released his cock and steadied his finger inside me. Our eyes met again and mine pleaded, 'I want you now, fuck me please!' His eyes darkened in response and he caught his breath. I knew he wanted to, yet he made no move to release me from my standing position against the wall. 'I am so close to the edge, let me feel you inside me before I explode,' my eyes begged. He lowered his head and took my lips in his mouth so that I couldn't see his refusal. Be patient, I told myself, but couldn't form a coherent thought when he was kissing me like that! With his finger inside me, he began stroking my clit with his thumb and I felt my orgasm building. I desperately wanted to spread open my legs and clench his cock with my hot wet pussy. In my fantasies he'd been naked and I caressed his muscles with unbridled pleasure while he rose above me time and again, driving me to the brink. But in this moment it was not to be. My hand tightened around his cock and I stroked him as though he were fucking me. Our breathing and moaning meant we were both about to explode. James slowed his hand movements down to maximise the pleasure for me and I increased the pressure for him. Sliding two fingers inside me, James grabbed my ass with his other hand so that his wrist was putting even more pressure on my clit. I had to grab him with both hands as I came. My body spasmed involuntarily for ages and I sounded as though I were weeping. Feeling selfish, I reached for his cock to pleasure him as much as he had pleasured me, but James stopped me. 'Why?' I asked, using my voice for the first time that evening. 'Because I can't sleep with my clients. It's a sacking offence. If you pleasure me, I would feel that I had crossed the line and it would be difficult for us to work together after tonight.'

Releasing a deep breath I didn't realise I was holding, I gathered my things and left. I continued having aftershocks while walking towards my car as my clit was still quite swollen. I wasn't satisfied. I had come but I still wanted him desperately. I knew the only thing that would satisfy me was his cock inside me, fucking me hard. I'd be patient, my time would come.

Sara, age 20
Bisexual
Steady relationship, not live-in
No children
University student
Illinois, USA

The best sex I ever had happened with my boyfriend. After polishing off a bottle of champagne together, we made love. We were making out, and the clothes came off. He ran his hands over my whole body, then followed his hands with his lips, slowly down to my pussy, then used his tongue to pleasure me while playing with my nipples with his fingers. Once I started to get really hot, I got on top of him in reverse-cowgirl and leaned back, moving myself up and down his cock, while he used his fingers on my clit to bring me to orgasm. He followed soon after. Unfortunately, I don't often come during sex, so this is one of the few times I can remember that I actually did, and it therefore must count as the best sex I've had so far.

Tight-lacing corsets are a huge turn-on for me, whether I'm the one laced up or whether they're on someone else. In erotic fiction or films, I prefer women over men, despite only ever having had sexual encounters with men. The same things continue to turn me on, plus the comfort of being in a loving relationship. I wish I could be more imaginative, but so far my fantasies are pretty much limited to things I've personally experienced. I fantasise about my boyfriend a lot, especially when we're apart for long periods of time. I like to replay previous encounters with him in my mind, or imagine what will happen the next time we're together in bed.

Alison, age 43
Heterosexual
Live-in relationship/marriage
Graduate degree
English teacher
Malaysia and China

I've written my 'Thetis' fantasy as a short story.

By some miracle, you find you have some time to show me the yacht. You know I would like to see it, although I am much more interested in the places where you play, the engine rooms, even the bilge tanks, rather than the luxury spaces that most people enjoy.

You text me: 'You free? Come to port, something to show you!' For you, of course, I am free, and although I was having lunch in Poble Nou with some friends, I hop in a taxi and am with you in about thirty minutes. I'm not really dressed for a trip around a yacht, wearing that same yellow skirt with high heels that I wore to the Princess, and just a cream cardigan, buttoned up.

There are people about, still lots to be done, people doing whatever they do on boats, splicing main braces and heaving to, so when we meet we can only do the Spanish kiss on the cheek and there's absolutely no question of holding hands except, of course, when you help me over steps and other tricky manoeuvres like that.

I don't really know the layout of boats, so I can't really quite imagine the route. Maybe you can tell me, but we start on the decks, you showing me the Jacuzzi, empty, the sun lounge. We are aware that people are popping in and out of doors, but the desire between us is electric; we are smiling as I ask you ridiculous questions and you try hard to answer them so I can understand, only for me to ask you a really clever one to challenge you, which you like.

We go inside into the owner's rooms; here is it quieter, hushed, the air very still. Suddenly we start to talk more quietly, we stand closer, our bodies almost touching, as we walk around, you touching my shoulder, ostensibly to guide me; I rest my hand on your back, possibly for support. We just need to touch each other!

You throw open the owner's bedroom suite with a flourish, and we both burst out giggling. We know exactly what we'd like to do, and the knowledge that we can't is both tantalising and hilarious. You make some very lewd suggestions about the size of the bed, and I pretend to be offended and flounce off into the bathroom. You move in behind me, quickly closing and locking the door.

I am standing in front of the big mirror above the sink and you come up behind me, slowly; you put your arms around me and I lean back into you. Silence. It feels good at last to be so close to each other again. We can feel each other breathing deeply. You bend down and slowly kiss me on the side of the neck. I gasp, your lips, so sensual, so soft, gently caress my skin and with one hand you lift my hair and move your kisses to the back of my neck. I can see your head bent low in the mirror and I raise my hands to reach into your thick hair. With your other hand, you reach into my cardigan, softly stroking the skin of my chest and then my breasts until you reach a nipple; already hard, you gently caress it, and again I moan with deep deep pleasure and you smile happily.

I try to turn around, and beg you to kiss me on the lips, but you won't. You stand up straight and with both hands you undo my cardigan, watching your hands, watching my eyes in the mirror as you do so. I keep my eyes fixed on your eyes in the mirror, enjoying the sensations of your fingers on my flesh. Suddenly, with a quiet and gentle movement, you pull both breasts out of my bra, holding them in your hands, weighing them, as if they were some precious commodity. I lean back into you even more, pressing my body into yours, feeling something hard in my back. We both smile at each other. Again, I beg you to kiss me on the lips and again you say no! You are just enjoying watching your fingers caress my breasts and nipples, the hard feel of them, watching as a flush comes to my cheeks and chest.

You bend down again and kiss me gently on the shoulder and very slowly you slide to your knees, not once taking your hands away from my breasts. Without your body to support me, I have to rest myself against the marble unit, my breathing hard and heavy. Slowly, you move your hands down from my breasts to my waist, to my hips, down past my thighs to my knees, where you reach my skin. Your hands are hot, soft and hard on my legs, and it feels good.

Slowly, you move your hands back up my legs. I'm really having to support myself now; my legs are weak with desire and I know that I am hot and moist with excitement and that at any minute you're going to discover this, and I'm going to feel a little ashamed of how quickly you've managed to excite and arouse me.

You know I'm aroused; you have seen the light in my eyes and don't need to do any confirmatory explorations. But you know what you want to do, and with one swift movement you hook your fingers in the top of my tanga and bring them down to my ankles. 'What?' I cry, not sure whether to laugh or be cross.

'Step out of them,' you order.

I do so. I have no choice and you put them in the pocket of your boiler suit, turn around and walk out of the bathroom.

Damn you! I push myself back into my bra and button myself up and, although my legs are still trembling with excitement, I manage to follow you out and back into the suite.

So the tour continues, only this time whenever we go up any stairs you, being the gentleman, go last in case I should fall. And each time one of your hands reaches up into my skirt, sometimes you just hold my buttocks, sometimes you explore a bit deeper, sometimes a finger comes out glistening and wet and you taste it, meeting my eyes as you do so. You know exactly what you're doing to me, and you are loving every minute. You see my nipples grow even harder and the now-permanent flush on my cheeks and my pupils dilated with erotic arousal.

At last, the final door. You open it and immediately I recognise your cabin. You turn and lock the door. I stand there, partly excited, partly terrified ... well, mainly excited, but not really sure what you're going to do. I am almost at screaming pitch.

Gently, you push me over to the bed. You sit me down and kneel in front of me so our faces are at the same height. Taking my head in both your hands, you kiss me; at first it is gentle, slow, but very quickly it becomes something more urgent, deeper, more penetrating. I hold you so tight, it's so good to feel you this close, the softness of your lips, and hardness and softness of your tongue, your teeth; I have no feelings other than when our bodies are touching.

You break away and gently undo my cardigan again, slowly pushing it off my shoulders, then undo my bra, pulling it off and throwing it into a dark corner. You bury your head between my breasts, and I hold you there as you smell my skin. Taking both of my breasts in your hands, you squeeze them together until you can put both nipples in your mouth at once. It feels so good, and I cling onto you, my hands in your hair as I feel your teeth, gently but firmly, biting the soft dark flesh.

You don't want to stop this; it feels so good and you can feel how much it is exciting me, but eventually you stop and push me back onto the bed, my legs still hanging over the edge. You stop for a while and look at me, and I wonder what you are thinking, but I love the fact you're watching me, half naked on your bed. It seems as if you are deciding whether or not to take off my skirt. Eventually you decide yes, it will only get in the way. Unzipping it, you slide it off and throw it after the other clothes. Now you kneel back and, with your hands on my knees, you move my legs apart. Even you are surprised by how open and red and moist she is, the juices almost beginning to run down my legs. You place each of them on your shoulders and very slowly start to kiss and stroke my inner thighs.

I am moving, begging you silently to come closer, closer where it is hot and wet, but you don't want to rush this pleasure and slowly, very slowly, in total torture you move inwards. Finally you bring your hands to her lips and open them, at the same time bending your head, and, with a strong tongue, begin to lick her. It is somewhere between a scream and a moan, but the feeling is so intense, so powerful and so sublimely beautiful that I just don't know what to do! I raise my pelvis up to meet your tongue and, within a few minutes, I can feel muscles beginning to shake and contract. So can you, and to increase my pleasure you insert one, two, three fingers inside, gently exploring, seeing how my moans increase with your movements. By now I have no idea where your tongue ends and where I begin, where your fingers meet your tongue with a bit of me in between them, a bit that is just a raging red fire of pleasure. I am terrified by these feelings; it has gone beyond just a mere physical sensation into something I could lose myself in, and I reach down and touch you. 'Don't stop,' I say, 'please, please, please do not stop.'

And you don't.

Until, some minutes later, the aftershocks still coursing through my body, you raise yourself up beside me so that I can cling to you. You stroke my hair and kiss my forehead as I, incapable of coherent speech, mumble something you can't quite understand. And you hold me tightly, so so tightly until my breathing has calmed down, and I look up at you, deep into your eyes, smelling my smell on your face, and I kiss you very gently on the lips and say, 'Thank you.'

To be continued ...

C, age 39
Heterosexual
Live-in relationship/marriage
Children
Bachelor's degree
Freelance writer/Photographer/stay-at-home mom
Maryland, USA

I rely on the same fantasy, much of the time. I am masturbating, and my husband stands next to the bed, also masturbating, until he comes on my face. It doesn't sound like much, but it is, shall we say, reliable.

Amber, age 24
Bisexual
Live-in relationship/marriage
No children
Some college
Sales
Texas, USA

My husband is a turn-on for me, as are compliments, some forms of role-playing, silky clothes and bubble baths. To be honest, anything can be sexy if I think about it the right way. I have two fantasies, the first one involves seducing a priest. That's fairly straightforward. The second is about my best friend. He says all the right things and makes all the right noises. There's nothing special about the fantasy. It changes. The most important thing is, he wants me and that *want* drives me crazy. It translates itself into me doing all sorts of dirty things in earnest. I fantasise about things being simple and hot, I guess.

Tiffini, age 34
Heterosexual
Virgin
Single, occasionally sexually active
College degree
Design
West Virginia, USA

I'm turned on by intelligence, someone to talk to. I think it's good to have some form of fantasy in any relationship, just don't go overboard or it could become chaos; remember simplicity. And yes, I'm a virgin, but that doesn't mean I'm innocent. I just haven't fallen in love with someone to have sex with. But I've had fun without 'going all the way'. The best sex I ever had was when I was in a nightclub with a boyfriend (now my ex-boyfriend) and went down on him in a corner. On the way back home we were walking along and found an empty area down a little slope of a hill and he went down on me (while I was gazing up at the stars).

In my fantasy there's a tall man with dark hair, not necessarily what mainstream society would consider good-looking.

He will do anything I want. He starts by undressing me gently and slowly, one item of clothing at a time. While doing so, he lets me undress him at the same time. He then lays me down and we make love, with him on top, and then me on top. We will be as one when he enters me and this continues on going, with different positions and not a lot of talking – we just let our bodies go in whatever direction is happening at the moment. Anything goes, a little spanking of me when I'm on top, a little of tying me to the bed when I'm on the bottom. When I climax I let him know how appreciative I am ... a little bit of petting and sucking and massaging.

Brenna, age 38
Heterosexual
Live-in relationship/marriage
Children
Bachelor's degree and professional certificate
Author/Teacher
Massachusetts, USA

The best sex I ever had was make-up sex when my husband and I got back together after being legally separated. We'd separated because he was having an affair. I had a fling of my own (a gent that was in an open relationship). While that didn't go well, badly enough that I decided I wasn't cut out for meaningless sex, it showed me that I was desirable again. To boot, I lost about 30 pounds, since I couldn't eat or sleep early on in the separation. I got my self-image up and found my muse again. I wasn't taking any crap from him. And, when we did end up in bed again, it was positively explosive. You see ... even my sister admits the man is my soul mate, so when we are together and doing well, we really mesh. There's also a deep emotional bond between us. The second best sex I've had was when he graduated boot camp. We'd been apart for eight weeks, and when we got back to my hotel room, the first time involved flying clothing and sex that was over – quite explosively for both of us – in about 90 seconds. We had sex, as memory serves, six times in the first thirty-six hours. Even later in our marriage, we averaged sex every eighteen hours, when he was in port. What would improve my sex life now would be me losing about 40 or more pounds and the kids being out more during times when we're both at home.

In the past I particularly enjoyed some of the old romance books, the ones that would be classified as soft bodice-rippers. The man is intent on the woman he wants. She is not entirely happy with the idea of being married to him, but she's drawn to him and seduced by him in all ways, and in the end they are together happily. He's always a very alpha-male type, and he's very protective and caring about the lady in his life. To be honest, this sort of seduction was always more stimulating to me than just seeing naked male bodies. I'm still turned on by alpha males. I think there are only a couple of other men that turn me on . . . ones that are clearly not alphas. I like attitude – not disrespect but attitude; not necessarily bad boys but not doormats, to be sure. I like men that are focused on me when they are with me. If they are checking out every other woman out there, they can forget a second date. They can talk to me . . . to my face, looking in my eyes. If they are talking to the chest (especially the chest, since I have a fairly impressive one), they are done for. I've met men who couldn't look at me and talk at the same time, because I had the nursing breasts and was wearing wench garb. I love eyes, intense, how the colours change, the expressions in them. I like intelligent men. I like men with a sense of humour, even if it's dark humour . . . sarcasm and irony.

I adore a certain amount of bondage, toy play – more

male-led than me leading, though I don't consider myself a sub. I have some recurring themes and some breakout fantasies. The recurring themes often involve a man intent on me, sweeping me away into hot sex, sometimes in places that I wouldn't normally consider having sex in real life. Obviously he's an alpha. My breakout fantasies are often things that my characters are experimenting with or doing. It might not be something I personally would do in real life (including same-sex experimentation), but if I can empathise with the character, I can certainly fantasise about it myself.

There is a man, the *only* other man I've considered marrying besides my husband. He's not much of an alpha and never has been. When my husband and I were separated, we came close to starting something, but he didn't want to be a rebound. He gave me time to decide, and I ended up back with my husband, so nothing ever happened between us . . . not even a kiss. In the fantasy I've lost my husband and we get a second chance together. He's hungry, because he's tired of waiting and won't give me the chance to change my mind again. His hunger gives him just that edge of alpha to him and the sex is often and explosive. Since I have few consensual things I don't do, you can pretty much vary it from there to just about everything a healthy, experimental hetero couple does in bed.

Name withheld, age 41
Heterosexual
Live-in relationship/marriage
No children
National Vocational Qualification
Not employed
Southwest England, UK

Watching women have sex with each other turns me on massively – to the point where I thought I was bi. However, never in my adult life have I met a woman I fancied or even really thought about outside of watching a porno. I think the reason I like it is that it concentrates on clitoral stimulation. Interestingly, answering this question has just made me realise that I never have the urge to write about it either.

At the moment Keanu Reeves is floating my boat; previously it was Ricky Martin. Straight sex is pretty much as wild as my imagination gets. Being fucked hard is the main focus usually. I tend to remember scenes from movies I've seen; I have a few faves – and I don't need to insert myself into them to enjoy thinking about them, I'm happy just to remember them.

I think I have given up on the idea of a competent lover. That sounds harsh but I mean someone who'll put their ego to one side long enough to learn what is basically a technique that will improve the more you practice it. I enjoy sex alone more than with another person these days. I always know sex is not going to live up to the hype, but I still live in hope. Things might improve if I could find a new man who is driven by sexual desire rather than inhibited by a fear of being too 'open' – a man who doesn't find my sexual confidence intimidating. Losing some weight would help me feel confident enough to throw myself around a bit more too.

My fantasies are very run of the mill and I have done a few of them – sex in a public place, picking up a stranger, etc. Sex with a woman was something I considered going to another city to try once (visit a gay bar maybe?) but I know that most lesbians are very masculine and therefore not the kind of women that have turned me on in films. Having said that, I never look at a very attractive woman and wonder if she's gay, so I don't think it's something I particularly want to have happen. I have a very strong libido – just the thought of the orgasm I'll have is sufficient to make me want to have sex. I'll often fantasise to help it along, but it will happen anyway. I write a lot of the things I like into my stories, so it's hard to pinpoint a particular fantasy – these often arouse me as I write them. I think the themes tend to be men who are totally hot for the heroine – who pursue them relentlessly. I know from my own personal experience that penetration isn't enough for female orgasm, so I often have the man add stimulation of the clitoris, or have the woman do it herself as part of the sex. I also love the thought of penetration with a finger while receiving oral sex; most of my male characters know to do this.

Sarah, age 31
Heterosexual
Live-in relationship/marriage
Children
College
Homemaker
West Midlands, UK

I'm turned on by men I can't have! Bad guys, but bad guys who are respectful to women, such as Tony Soprano from the HBO television show, Robbie Williams, Colin Farrell (he's so sexy), men who work outside (they wear riggers and have big rough hands). Men in suits are OK as long as they are in charge. I cannot be doing with men who wear make-up or spend time on their hair.

The best sex I ever had happened a few years ago, I think I was 22 at the time. Someone at work had been showing me a lot of attention and being very flirty. He was involved with someone (he ended up marrying her), but it was like the forbidden fruit – I wanted what I couldn't have. Anyway, he gave me a lift home and asked me to call him. I said no, he knew where I was if he wanted me. Later that night he knocked on my door and before I had even closed it we were at it. I had a nightdress on and he lifted it, pulled my panties aside and fucked me up against my front door. It was passionate, but rough. His hands were big; he was a lot taller than me and heavily built. He just knew what to do, exactly where to touch me and kiss me, and we had the most amazing night. He was very well-endowed and I felt every single thrust. I had never had sex other than in the missionary position until that night. No one had ever gone down on me or entered me from behind. He pulled my hair when he was behind me and it was such a turn-on. He opened me up with his fingers and thumbs and went down on me and I came so hard and fast. He just kept on going and never stopped, making sure I was enjoying it as much as him. (I'm getting turned on just remembering this.) The best thing other than the sex was that he didn't look down on me afterwards, we both knew it was a one-night thing and we still get on great now; although I no longer work with him I see him around occasionally. He's always nice to me and I'll always think of that night as the best I've ever had. I think if I was ever tempted to have an affair it would have to be with him.

I think my fantasies have stayed the same as when I was younger. I have romantic fantasies that some big strapping man is going to sweep me off my feet and then fuck me senseless! However, my favourite fantasy is to go down on a woman. I would like to make a woman come with my tongue. I'd know exactly how and what to do because, let's face it, most men just don't have a clue. Watching women really really turns me on – blonde women who are slim and have small breasts with soft pink nipples.

The Romantics

Kitten, age 20
Bisexual
Live-in relationship/marriage
High School
Unemployed
South Wales, UK

The gentleness of the female form has always turned me on; for the men it's the knight in shining armour thing. I fantasise several times a day, usually about a dark, handsome, mysterious stranger taking advantage of me. My favourite fantasy starts with my best friend approaching me while we're out with a group of mates partying up a mountain. We sit around chatting for a while, then as we drink more we get everyone to play a game of hide and seek. As this game is being played, my best mate finds me. I run and he chases me, finally catching me, and we fall to the ground near the top of this mountain. The fog is rolling around us on the ground and the moon is full and the stars are out, and we look at each other for a minute, then we kiss gently, slowly getting more passionate until we're ripping each other's clothes off and rolling around in the dewy grass under the stars and moon ... well, use your imagination for the rest (it's very romantic, yet very passionate).

Barbara, age 58
Heterosexual
Single, occasionally sexually active
Master's degree
Artist
California, USA

I'm turned on by tender intellectuals who are curious and playful and not afraid to experiment, but who know when to stop. I think I used to fantasise about being raped; I thought it would be a way to have sex but not take responsibility for my feelings. This was the attitude of a scared child. I no longer have this fantasy, but enjoy participating in my own sexual experience. Now I just play and have a great time. I also fantasised about being covered with whipped cream, though found the experience to be lacking; it melts too quickly. I have fulfilled my fantasies, and found some better than others. I let go of the ones that did not feel good to me.

My fantasy begins with skinny-dipping. The water feels so good. We then sit in a tub and draw on each other with water-soluble utensils, followed by washing each other all over. When dry, I would be tickled all over with feathers, then laid down in front of the fire, where honey would be dripped all over my front. My lover then licks the honey off and kisses me all over, turning me over and fucking me front and back (not in the asshole, though – I've tried it and it just hurts without pleasure).

Breezy, age 30
Bisexual
Live-in relationship/marriage
No children
Some college
Retail Manager
Illinois, USA

I have been sexually aware since I was a child. The first thing I saw was a copy of *Playboy* magazine. I remember thinking I wanted to be her and have her. Then, as I got older, sex became more of a way to feel things. I was closed off emotionally and yet through sex I was able to really be me. I love lace, silk and satin. And I have had many older men as lovers. I guess I wanted to learn as much as possible. I find athletic people turn me on. I love beautiful legs and devastating smiles. I'm a sucker for American Football players.

In my fantasy we are in a field having a picnic on a perfect sunny day. Suddenly from out of nowhere my fantasy man grabs me and lowers me to the ground. He kisses me deeply, taking my breath away. I gasp as he starts to kiss my neck, moving lower and lower. I suddenly realise that he has been undressing me and is slowly taking his tongue down my body, first over my nipples, then down my stomach, lower and lower until he comes to the apex between my thighs.

I moan as he slowly brings me to a roaring climax. It starts to darken and I realise there are raindrops falling on us. But he feels so good that I do not stop him. I come again and again. He slowly starts to move back up my body with his tongue, kissing me deeply and plunging into me at the same time.

There is thunder now. The rain is coming down harder and faster. He feels incredible. I start to come yet again and I feel him starting to as well. Neither of us notices the weather any more, it is all about each other. We both have incredible orgasms and lie there next to each other for a few moments, taking in everything that has happened.

Then we go for round two.

Sarah, age 47
Bisexual
Live-in relationship/marriage
No children
Postgraduate qualification
Writer/Teacher
Norfolk, UK

For me the best sex is waking up in the morning feeling my lover pressing against me, turning to him, stroking, kissing, fondling, his mouth on my breasts, my hand sliding down to his cock, imagining him entering me, then him entering me, getting smooth inside, then sliding, then frantic, pushing my pelvis against his, feeling his back buck, feeling my insides slicked, then sliding over onto my side, pressing my thighs against him, him entering again, feeling the tight port stretch for him while he strokes my shoulders, then again, and we end with my hands and my mouth around his cock and hot juice rolling down my belly between us.

The things that turn me on are my partner, trees, the sea, wind blowing across the beach or fields, stones from the beach. I like to fantasise about making love on the beach, in the dunes, in fields, along footpaths. This recurs whenever we are walking on the beach, in fields, or along footpaths.

Ruthie, age 22
Heterosexual
Live-in relationship/marriage
Bachelor's degree
Singer/Songwriter
Florida, USA

When I was way younger, I used to fondle my girlfriends; that was erotic. They used to do it to me too. I love black men with dreadlocks who smoke marijuana. That's the only turn-on in men. In women, I'm turned on by the need for intimacy and also creativity, a love of music and poetry – an appreciation for life in its totality. In my fantasy I see myself with a gorgeous woman ... slender, sexy, delicious ... not there just to fuck me, but to bond with me spiritually and emotionally. I want to make love to her in every way – and I want her to knock my senses out of my head.

Name withheld, age 19
Heterosexual
Virgin
Steady relationships, not live-in
Nursing student
Unknown, USA

My boyfriend always manages to turn me on, and also reading Black Lace novels, because I find it better to imagine everything than seeing it on TV or online. I used to feel uncomfortable just thinking about sex, but now, not so much. I've become more comfortable with my sexual thoughts. I don't really have a place to have sex yet; I don't want to have to sneak it in before anyone gets home, and I want to feel like I am definitely ready to have sex.

My favourite fantasy thus far has been when I imagine my boyfriend and me having sex in the middle of a park, surrounded by all these beautiful flowers, in the middle of the night, under the stars. I am on top.

Carrie, age 34
Homosexual
Single, occasionally sexually active
Children
College
Federal government employee/Photographer/Writer (at heart)
Ontario, Canada

I wrote my fantasy to a friend on Facebook:

soaking in the tub for hours
you've got me touching myself
thinking, 'what'd she do in the shower?'

fantasising: you here with me in my bath
picturing that coy laugh
... then your unintended sigh
as i sink down between your ...

no – stop! that's too fast! that's not right ...

start over ...

i close my eyes ...
my hand goes there ...
dreaming about being with you
dreaming about you here

is there somethin'
to the fact that we've gotten to talking?
(don't worry girl, i ain't into stalking)
i'm thinking, 'well ... maybe it's a sign ...'

open your eyes to a hot reality
just maybe this could be
the introduction of things to come ...
inclinations of slow seductions,
visions of us as one

wrinkly in the tub after hours
wishing you were closer
just so i could watch you in the shower

i imagine you:
whispering my name . . .
one step forwards,
curtain drawn . . .

suddenly the room's feeling warmer

there's you, back arched
holding on, up against the corner

i see you touching
playing between there
and i can't help but stare

one step closer,
my clothes are wet
you haven't even noticed me yet
you're so deep into you
steam's rising off you . . .

water's feeling warmer
(or maybe it's just you)
steam blurring my view
don't know where to start
i just know i need to be next to you

again, i hear you whisper my name
more of me . . . wet
i'm feelin' myself pulsing
i'm a throbbing, soaking wreck . . .
'n i haven't even touched you yet

you turn to face me

moisture dripping down your . . .
i resist every urge to kneel and taste . . .

innocently enough . . .
i begin
with a kiss . . .

melting . . .
i feel the gentle sway forwards of your hips
and your hands reaching for my . . .

Name withheld, age 24
Heterosexual
Celibate
No children
Graduate student
Teacher
California, USA

I enjoy fantasising about having good vivid sex with a few orgasms; celebrity sex with Colin Farrell, Jonathan Rhys Meyers and Henry Cavill; and anal sex. My ex brought it up and got me so turned on and interested in it. I would love a man to fill me there but gently, lovingly.

In my fantasy my lover and I are seeing each other. It's our first night and we go to his place and he seduces me. He covers my body with kisses and licks, sucking and kissing me until he licks me clean. He won't let me touch him though. Then he makes sweet, passionate love to me. Later, after a warm bath, he seduces me into letting him take me anally. Slowly. Sweetly.

A Blast from the Past

Trudy, age 25
Heterosexual
Live-in relationship/marriage
Children
A levels
Homemaker/Care assistant
Northamptonshire, UK

I like men who have passion for what they do, so I kind of get aroused when a man is shouting when something he really cares about gets mucked up by someone, even if it's me who's getting shouted at. It's safe to say I could never work for Gordon Ramsay. I would be too turned on all the time. Historical themes turn me on, mainly Regency going back to Tudor, some modern day. (I did historical re-enactment.) Add to this bodices, castles, vampire films, i.e. *Dracula* or *Interview with a Vampire*, and tall moody men. I still like the bodices; I have a nice collection of them now. My husband figures in my fantasies quite a bit. If we go away together we make sure the hotel is old and has a huge four-poster bed to get the history into it.

Lindsay, age 23
Bisexual
Live-in relationship/marriage
College degree
Customer Service Advisor
South Wales, UK

My main early sources of inspiration were the numerous 'slash' or gay fiction websites. I lived vicariously through other people's sex lives – not just the hardcore 18-rated things, but the build-up, the romance, the arguments, the passion. It drew me in. At the same time I had begun to appreciate fine underwear and started to get interested in fetish from a clothing point of view, realising the huge sexual and sensual promise in fabrics like leather, PVC and velvet. The touch of them on my skin was enough to arouse me.

I'm still reading gay fiction, though I now read a broader field of erotica. I have also kept an interest in the world of fetish, including tight-lacing corsets, vintage clothes, and bondage. Although I rarely manage to go to fetish clubs, the feeling of being someplace where people will appreciate your corseted silhouette and PVC-clad thighs brings an incredible erotic thrill. I have occasionally been a Mistress to some very close friends, and their devotion to me is highly erotic. For some reason I also have an unhealthy fixation on hot tubs, though I'm yet to experience their fullest promise.

At first I was very confused about my sexual feelings towards both men and women – I assumed there was something wrong with me! As such, I was a late bloomer and did not lose my virginity until the age of nineteen. When I first became sexually aware, I found it difficult to touch myself and bring myself to orgasm without the aid of a vibrator. I was not very in tune with what turned me on and how to enjoy myself. As I have come to accept my sexual preferences I have found it easier to express myself in all ways, and am certainly more attuned to my own body. It's like I'm more comfortable in my own skin. I am now in a committed relationship. My partner satisfies me fully, but there are some fantasies, involving more people, that I will now never be able to fulfil. I sometimes regret I did not have a more wild life before I settled down! But I am still able to enjoy several aspects of my sexual fantasies, like attending burlesque and fetish clubs, and dressing in a manner that thrills me. I enjoy a very healthy sex life with my partner, though I don't have much bondage or fetish included, certainly not as much as before I met him. He satisfies me in other ways, and is always willing to try new things, but there's always room for improvement; life would be boring otherwise!

Generally my fantasies involve me being somewhere I will never go: for example, a far-off planet, an ocean liner in the 1930s, an ancient jungle kingdom. There I meet people from contemporary media – shameful, I know, mixing my fantasies! They variously indulge my whims with me and people of my choosing. However, a very different recurring fantasy involves me in heavy bondage, unable to see, but feeling several people doing various things to me, and I'm powerless to resist (as if I would want to!). I imagine that it's different people every time. I must be dominant and submissive.

Currently my favourite fantasy takes place in Victorian times. I am a glamorous courtesan – think Nicole Kidman in *Moulin Rouge*, but with more cleavage! My 'client' is a masked man with long, slightly greying hair and a sultry Scottish drawl. This, I am sure, stems from my near obsession with Denis Lawson. He is at first prim and proper until a tango begins to play and we have the raunchiest dance, gradually ripping off layers of stiff Victorian clothing until our breath is ragged and I am in just a corset and dainty boots, and he just in silk bloomers. I can feel his firm body against me, his hard cock. It doesn't matter that the room is full of other courtesans and their partners, I'm enjoying giving them a show! I kneel before him and offer to taste him, suck him. He catches my hand as I move to slide down his bloomers and pulls me up roughly, saying all he wants now is to complete the act we have been dancing around for the last hour and make me feel him hard inside me. This new-found manliness turns me to jelly every time. He shoves me roughly against the wall and does well on his promise, taking me hard, licking and nipping at my ears and throat. I can see over his shoulder other couples and groups taking the initiative. He pulls my corset free at last and, as he bites and laps at my nipples, I just can't contain myself any more and come so hard.

Julia, age 42
Heterosexual
Live-in relationship/marriage
Children
College
Teacher
Essex, UK

I realised I was very interested in men by about the age of fourteen. I used to be mad on soldiers and always found hairy chests attractive. I knew you couldn't do anything about it, since girls back then didn't. I've always loved uniforms, especially police uniforms. I love the idea of play-acting – police and culprit, fire and rescue, that sort of thing – and even did some tying up, which was great fun. I still love uniforms and hairy men. I love rugby players; I'm married to a 6'4" one, but the changing-room scenario is exciting. I love men together, find that very exciting – firemen, soldiers, policemen, customs officers and men in prison. If I could break that in, it would be very nice.

I used to fantasise like mad about all different ideas, but most men I've met don't really like it much and some have laughed and said, 'I'm not doing that!' I have found sex is far less satisfactory now than when I was young; it's a real disappointment. I've had to dampen down my libido to non-existent, which saddens me a lot. My imagination has had to take a back seat; even sex toys scare men, so you can't share the experience. Having some time to play around, getting my other half to lighten up, would improve my sex life. We've not had sex for two years, and I gave up long ago, it's all solo these days. I would like to fulfil at least one of my fantasies. A lot of these fantasies my husband could easily do, but he will not.

In my fantasies I always go in for historical or period costumes. Usually I'm mistress of a large seventeenth-century house, and I go out one hot night and come across the groom in the stables, where he's half-naked either washing or lying back on the hay. These can take place in various centuries and take all forms: maid, farmer, lord and variations, rather like *Poldark* and *Pride and Prejudice* but much hotter. I go through Tudor, Victorian – all the eras! The groom fantasy is my top one and has been for a long time. I can start it very quickly, and continue it in chapters, adding more detail each time. It's often set in early Victorian days.

The house I live in is very large and remote, and the whole place feels repressed. I came here to be governess to an older couple's child and the mother has since gone, leaving me as a companion to a withered-up old lady who sleeps a lot. The husband is old and reads or sleeps, so life is not very exciting. All the household staff have aged with their owners except me. I'm dark-haired, with my dress buttoned up to the neck, but have a full figure and very large breasts. I have to contain all this in a prim dark dress. At night I take off the outer layers and wander the house with a candle looking for something: life, passion, feeling. My nightdress is thin and white and my hair long and loose as I go from room to room longing for something: to be touched, to feel the heat of a man. I know that this is what I need, but there's no outlet for it. I go to the library and get down a book I found by accident many months ago. It's old and worn and the writing is in French. I know what it contains as I have found it many times before. The book is full of old etchings showing men and women in various positions. The women are from another century; their gowns are lifted up and men are between their legs, licking the orgasmic-looking women. Other pictures have a woman with big breasts hanging out from an unbuttoned dress while two men suck her nipples as a third man plays with her. The pictures I love most are the ones of men lying, alone in the countryside or in their study, lazily stroking their cocks or alternatively rubbing them hard. I look and look, I can't take my eyes off them. I want to see and feel one. I want it inside me with the weight of a man holding me down and doing the things that the women are doing in my book. To look at this drives me mad and makes the pain of my frustration worse. My only outlet is objects. The library has a small staircase with a low wooden finial shaped like an acorn, and by climbing over it horse style I can get the wooden acorn to enter me. I ride this up and down to ease the urgency. Afterwards, I take various items with me and, when I'm back in my bed, I lie down and let the wind from the open window play over me, using the objects one by one while rubbing and squeezing my breasts and imagining if only . . . This has become a nightly occurrence, and the longing gets worse.

The big house has a large separate stable block with a small living area inside. I often include this in my walk, stopping to feed and stroke the horses, then go on my way. The current groom is a really ugly man who, by great luck, has found himself an equally ugly woman to marry and they are planning to move away. This character is called Hilton, and he takes great delight in shocking me and making lewd comments whenever I go near the stables. He's so repulsive it means nothing to me, but this day he tells me that he has a stud horse of fine quality to breed with one of our mares and asks if I'd care to watch. I feign uninterest, but secretly I'm curious and I go with him to the stable.

The atmosphere inside is strange. It smells of sweat and steam and of a strange kind of excitement. The mare is reluctant and backs off as she's cornered by the stud horse. Hilton looks on leering, telling me that, although they are animals, it's exciting. I pretend to be disgusted and turn on my heel to walk away, though I want to watch it all. But Hilton's face and the atmosphere make me want to leave. In the days that follow I hear Hilton has finally left and a new groom has moved into the stable. Apparently he's very good with horses and expected to do well, being Romany. I know a little about the Romany and feel excited that a man of mystery is in the stable. They tell me his name is Jack, and I imagine that he's probably as old as everyone else.

One hot night I feel more than usually unsettled. It's spring; the woods around the house are alive again, and everywhere there's love and sex, but not for me. The night is so warm I get no comfort indoors so I go outside to take a walk to the lake. My gown is wet against my body, and I walk on the soft grass down into the woods. As I pass the stable block, I hear horses whinnying and see a light in the windows, although it's late. Out of curiosity, I go over and look through the window. In the candlelit stable I see horses and a man thrashing about. Wanting a better view, I slip through the open door, a convenient beam becoming a good place to hide and peer out from. The scene unfolds like a dream: the groom Jack is the most beautiful man I've ever seen. He's tall, well over six feet, and has shoulder-length dark hair. His face is very masculine, with dark stubble, his shoulders broad. Dark hair spills down his chest, ending in a delightful trickle into loosely belted trousers. He's sweaty, he's dirty, and he looks magnificent. He's getting two horses to mate but is much more successful than Hilton as the mare is willing. The stud mounts the mare and I gasp in amazement at the size of his cock. As the stud services the mare, Jack keeps up his encouragement. The air is so highly charged you can taste it. The servicing goes on for some time, and I see a change in Jack's face. His eyes blaze; he runs his hand through his hair and looks agitated – or is it excited? – as the horse comes down.

Jack turns to wash his arms and hands. As he rubs the soap over his body, his movements become more deliberate. He runs it over his stomach and to the edge of his belt, then he suddenly drops the soap, walks over to a pile of hay bales and lazily lies back against them. I sigh, and he looks over; maybe he heard me, I'm not sure. Jack continues to rub over his chest and stomach with one hand, then with the other he undoes the buckle of his belt and opens the first two buttons, releasing a big and very hard cock. He pulls down his trousers and in the candlelight traces he grasps it in his hand and, after some very slow strokes, begins to move his hand faster. The act becomes frantic and I watch in awe as this magnificent man pleasures himself. After what seems quite a long time, he groans in a gentle, low way and comes over his stomach. By this time I feel faint with desire, but I don't want to move and break the spell.

Jack stands up after some time and washes his body, drying himself with handfuls of sweet hay. He makes himself a bed among the sacks and straw and half covers himself with a rough blue blanket, dimming his lantern. Not knowing what to do, I stand there hiding, wanting to go to him as he lies back with his arms behind his head. There's a movement and I see that his cock is aroused again, and Jack calls out, 'I know you are there. I have watched you. I have stood outside your window wanting you, I have followed you and had to stop myself from taking you then and there in the woods and by the lake and everywhere you've been!' He then pulls back the blanket and I walk over to him. I kneel down and he rips off my flimsy gown, lifts my hair up and buries his face into my neck, kissing me passionately.

J, age 25
Heterosexual
Virgin
Celibate
University degree
Marketing Executive
Scotland, UK

Being a randy little madam, anything used to turn me on. I especially liked lesbian things (which continues somewhat today) and the whole teacher and pupil scenario. I enjoyed watching porn and reading anything with a little sex in it. As soon as I was old enough I was reading those bodice-rippers that do have some nice sex in them, then moved onto bigger and better things as I got older. I still like to watch porn (especially rough and ready sex, lesbian sex, group sex and pure fantasy films). I also enjoy reading erotic stories. I take things that have happened through my boring workdays and change their outcome so that we all get some good sex, which is always a turn-on when I see their boring selves the next day in the office and they have no idea what I've been thinking of.

I am still technically a virgin, but, as I've grown up, I've found myself less bothered by how much I fantasise and what I fantasise about. I have developed from just reading a story or watching a film to fantasising about what I would have liked to see happen, so I'm becoming more sexually confident – strange but true. And I know what I like and have no problems with demanding it – if only I could find a decent, good-looking rich man to give it all to me! The only thing that holds me back is the lack of a decent man/decent men. I have never even found someone that I could use for a little while. If they're sweet and cute then I walk all over them and if they're self-confident then they know their own worth and only go for big-titted, common sluts – dammit all to hell! If I found a man I would have no problem with sharing/acting out all my fantasies with him. And then sharing his! So long as I trusted him then anything's possible.

One of my current favourite fantasies is that of an early nineteenth-century lady who lives in a house with her parents. One night the butler (who's a slightly older man than her) catches her trying to sneak a man into her room and basically, to cut a long story short, bribes her into sucking him off to prevent him from telling her parents of her behaviour. She is a novice, untutored, and he teaches her what she should do. After that, the pair find ways to be together when the house is empty. They fuck on the doorstep, on the stairs, in the servant's quarters, in her bed, her parent's bed, and against a lot of walls. Lots of really hot, deep, sweaty sex – nothing sweet and pure! I think I like the whole reverse-role thing where the submissive person is actually the person in the dominating position, and I am a fan of bodice-ripper scenes. The actual fantasy/storyline changes each time, but I do like to have fun with it. It's like dress-up for my mind!

Nicola, age 30
Heterosexual
Single, occasionally sexually active
Children
College student
Manchester, UK

I enjoy fantasising about inexperienced younger men to whom I teach lots of rude things, or geeky guys who don't think anyone could find them attractive, but under their glasses and nerdy clothes is a buff, sexy man with great stamina. I now know that my imagination and experiences don't have to involve me just pleasuring the man and not receiving pleasure. More often than not I get it all and they get little or none. I would love to be a dominatrix.

Here is my fantasy. I am a mixed race, big and beautiful princess in Georgian times and I live with my parents and two younger brothers in a country house, since my naval officer husband was lost at sea. My father doesn't like me being lonely, so he asks his younger naval captain friend to marry me. I like the captain; he's friendly and kind and very handsome. In the drawing room one evening the captain and I are having a conversation after everyone has retired to bed. He says he's going away for a few weeks and is happy to be marrying me because I make him very aroused, and he tells me that he'd like it if I were his madam and would I please punish him. He adds that he has to be dominating in his job, so he wants me to dominate him. I find this really exciting and decide to play along. I tell him that I'm going to punish him for looking at my big breasts while we were dining and I instruct him to bend over the table with his trousers down and his bottom in the air. While he's doing this, I get my riding crop. I position myself to the side of him and spank him with it, soft at first, then harder. I'm really getting a thrill, and he's so excited that when I let him stand up he spurts come all over my dress. I make him get on his hands and knees and lick it off, which he does obediently. I tell him that he must come to see me tomorrow for more punishment.

The next day I again meet up with the captain in the drawing room, where it's quiet. He says he has been thinking about me all day and that he couldn't sit down for hours because I whipped him very well, adding that if there's anything he can do for me then I should let him know. I nod my head and tell him I'm very angry that he enjoyed what I did and that I'll have to punish him harder today for enjoying it so much. He has an excited glint in his eye, but pretends to be very sorry. I pick up my riding crop and instruct him to strip. He takes off all his clothes and folds them, placing them neatly on the nearest chair, which I find quite sweet. He then stands naked and erect in the middle of the room.

I walk slowly around my fiancé studying every part of him, paying careful attention to his long legs, lean body and firm buttocks with its faint pink lines. Looking at these lines that I'd made only yesterday makes me very aroused. I'm aware that he feels uncomfortable being so closely scrutinised, but that only makes me more excited. I walk up behind him and whisper in his ear for him to get on his hands and knees atop the desk so I can see him better. He does so tentatively, trying hard not to show his excitement. I can see his balls hanging down; I tap them lightly with my riding crop and hear a sharp intake of breath, so I tap them harder and harder. The captain tells me that if I keep doing that he will come. I say that he's not to talk to me and that he is only to come when I say so. He nods and lowers his head, and I whip him on his bottom hard to show him I'm his boss. He whimpers, which drives me to whip him again and again, causing three angry red lines to appear on his behind. I tell him to lie on his back, and when he does his dick points right up to the ceiling. I stroke the riding crop slowly up and down his hard shaft and see his balls tighten, telling me that he's ready to come. He tries to touch his cock, but I hit his hands away, reminding him that I will tell him when he's allowed to come. But I myself am so aroused at the control I have that it's all I can do to stop myself from lifting up the skirts of my dress and lowering myself onto his hard rod. He looks into my eyes and I can see that he's at his limit so I tell him, 'OK, Captain, give it your best shot', and at this he shoots his load straight up into the air with a loud groan. He has come all over himself and I tell him to clean himself up. While he's doing so, I walk over to the chair on which he carefully placed his clothes earlier. I take his hanky out of his pocket, lift up my skirts, spread my legs, and wipe the hanky between my pussy lips until a big, wet, sweet-smelling stain appears. I replace the hanky just before the captain returns, still naked but clean. I sit on the edge of the desk and lift up my skirts, showing him my moist pussy. His eyes grow wide and his member grows hard again. I tell the captain to kneel between my legs, and he buries his face in my pussy, licking and nibbling my clit so well that he makes me come with such a force I nearly fall off the desk.

He rises to his feet and stands between my legs. I can feel his hardness pressing against my pussy lips. He leans forwards and whispers in my ear, 'I know it is wrong for me to take your innocence before we are married but I ask your permission to let me please you the way you please me.' He steps back, his eyes pleading, and I remind him that I was married before and that I would be honoured if he pleased me, so with a smile he slowly enters me. I wrap my arms around him and as he goes deeper I can feel my orgasm rise. The captain thrusts his solid member deeper and harder inside me and brings me to the most amazing orgasm I've ever had. As I come I feel him explode deep inside me.

After our breathing stabilises, the captain looks me in the eye and smiles, saying he is going to enjoy being married to me. I tell him he's allowed to get dressed, to which he bows, and that makes me smile. When the captain is fully dressed, he gives me a long passionate kiss and says he will miss me while he's away. As he walks out of the door, I tell him that if he misses me too much he can smell the hanky. Intrigued, he pulls out his hanky and smells it and, as he does, a huge smile spreads across his face.

Name withheld, age 44
Bisexual
Live-in relationship/marriage
Children
Master's degree
User-Interface Designer
California, USA

I mostly fantasise about being dominated, overwhelmed, manhandled, or otherwise forced into sexual situations. In these fantasies I am being lusted after madly and seduced, and occasionally being worshipped, or being the seducer of a sweet young thing. One of my long-time favourites is a classic Victorian romance-type fantasy. I'm a proper young lady in Victorian times (more or less), wearing a long elaborate gown with a plunging neckline. I've slipped away from a party and my chaperone to meet secretly with a young man – a handsome, fair young man whose family owns the estate where the party is being held. We've agreed to rendezvous in a quiet room, but he hasn't yet arrived. While I'm waiting for him, his good-for-nothing half-brother lets himself into the room and finds me there.

The half-brother is handsome in a dark, cruel, sneering way. He's bitter because he's older but has somehow been cheated out of his rightful place as his father's heir. When he sees me, he knows immediately what I'm doing here. He torments me a while with verbal fencing – I desperately want him to leave before his brother comes and our plans are revealed. He suggests he might tell my chaperone that he found me here, alone, clearly planning to meet some-one ... who?

I decide to bolt from the room, but he has locked the door. I turn back and find him standing there, too close to me. He tells me I'm really quite beautiful ... and starts stroking my hair, my neck ... I tell him to take his hands off me, I threaten to scream ... He asks if I want to explain to everyone why I'm here alone in this room with him in the first place.

I'm trying to decide what to do, but his hands are distracting me. He's holding me too close, now he's kissing my neck, moving down to my breasts ... I try to pull away, but he's holding me too tightly. Suddenly he throws me onto the sofa and looms over me. I try to struggle up, but I'm tangled in my gown and his weight is pressing down on me. His hands are everywhere, he's biting my neck and then, in a fit of passion, he tears open the front of my gown. I cry out but he covers my mouth with his ... I'm going liquid, I can't believe what's happening to me.

He chuckles; *he* knows what's happening. He says it's lucky he got to me first, his brother wouldn't know what to do with a girl like me. He lifts up my skirt, reaches underneath ... I beg him not to do it, but he won't listen, he won't stop ... and I'm not sure I really want him to. I threaten again to scream, and he asks if I want everyone to see me all exposed like this.

His hand is in a place that I don't even want to know I have, I'm melting, I'm panting, I don't know what's happening ... Then his hands are at his own waist and the next thing I know something is entering me Down There. I try to cry out but I'm coming ...

Knock, Knock ... Who's There?

Name withheld, age 43
Heterosexual
Single, occasionally sexually active
Some college
Executive Assistant
North Carolina, USA

My current fantasy is to have sex with a totally hot, tall, dark and handsome stranger. After strong passionate kisses, we will slowly undress each other, then he'll guide me over to the bed and lay me on my back. He takes off my panties and runs his hands over my pussy and sniffs me. He uses his fingers to open my lips and slowly licks my clit. He plunges his tongue deep inside me, tasting my juices and telling me how good I taste. My back is arched, and he puts his hand on my stomach and tells me to calm down because this is going to take a while. I claw at the sheets as I feel his tongue circling my clit and licking my lips hungrily. He pushes my legs up high and licks all the way down to my asshole. He licks and teases me by sticking his tongue in just a little way. He then asks me if I've ever had someone tongue-fuck my ass and I whisper no. He plunges his tongue in my ass and I can feel it slowly moving in and out. I'm dizzy with desire because this is so taboo but feels so good. He licks and sucks my hole and fingers my pussy. He pulls his fingers out and licks them and then starts devouring my clit and pussy again. I scream out loudly as he brings me to climax and he keeps on licking. I try to squirm away, but he grabs my thighs and pulls me back even closer to him and his darting tongue. He looks up and says, 'I told you this was going to take a while.' My body is covered in goose bumps and he starts in on what will be a wave of orgasms for me. He then flips me over and licks my ass from behind. I'm on all fours and trembling, his tongue hungrily slurping all the juice from my pussy. I arch my back and grind my ass into his face. He pulls back and says, 'Yes, baby . . . give that ass to me. Make me suck you and tongue you harder.' I explode again and I can feel the juices begin to run down my thighs . . . I feel his tongue licking anxiously after those juices and I cannot believe that I am being devoured like this. He is so hungry for every last drop and never takes his hands off me. He grips my ass and plunges his tongue deep inside me, sucking and moaning and slurping me . . . I can hardly take it. I scream out for him to fuck me . . . he says he won't yet. He works his way from my dripping cunt to my asshole and plunges his tongue inside me again. I'm shaking, I'm moaning and screaming and grasping at the sheets. I beg him to fuck me. He mounts me from behind and then stops. He pulls out and asks me to suck him. I scurry around like a dog in heat and take his hard veiny cock in my mouth. I hear him let out a long moan and he tells me how hot my mouth is and not to suck him to completion because he has other plans for the load he has inside him. I suck hungrily and I feel his hands running through my hair. He tells me how good my ass looks from that angle and I suck him even harder. I taste his sweet pre-come and I want more. He pushes me back and tells me not to be such a greedy girl. I smile and he pushes me back around onto my knees. I am breathing so heavily with the anticipation of his first thrust into me. He takes me and starts out slowly but very deeply. His cock feels amazing . . . like hard steel. He picks up his pace and stops momentarily to lick my pussy again to tell me how good it tastes and feels . . . I scream for him to fuck me harder. He plunges deep into me and grabs my ass tightly and he unloads his hot come inside me . . . I scream out and orgasm too. The thought of him driving into me drives me wild. He screams out my name and then pulls out and plunges his hard dripping cock into my ass. I gasp out loudly but love it. He pounds me hard and I come again. He stops and then gets on his knees and buries his face in my dripping pussy and eats me all over again.

Crystal, age 40
Heterosexual
Live-in relationship/marriage
Four-year college degree
Writer
New York, USA

I'm turned on by intelligent alpha males. The best sex I ever had was masturbating on the phone while my online pen pal did the same on the other end, and hearing him come at the same time I did as he said my name. My favourite fantasy is having sex for the first time with him – the man I write to daily online but have never met. My sex life would improve if I could finally fulfil my fantasies in real life with this man.

Rowan, age 40
Heterosexual
Live-in relationship/marriage
Children
College
Writer
New England, USA

I feel so much more comfortable with and proud of my sexuality. It's not only part of who I am, but part of my power as a woman. I believe that women who ignore their sexuality are not as powerful as they can be and have cut themselves off from a very important part of who they are. My sexuality is part of who I am, and my imagination only gets better with age and confidence.

Some of the best sex I ever had was when I met a lover at a hotel. He was dressed in a tux. The role-play was that he was the groom-to-be and I was a bridesmaid with the hots for him and wanted just one time with him before he married my friend. We fucked for well over an hour on that fantasy, pleasing each other orally, vaginally and anally. It was wonderful.

I like to fantasise about being a courtesan and pleasing men of my choice; being a goddess, worshipped and adored; and, surprise – seducing the package delivery boy! For some reason I find myself frequently feeling frisky in the early afternoons. My kids are in school, I'm home alone and my mind . . . wanders. Before I know it, I'm up in my bedroom masturbating. One of my favourite fantasies is that, before I get upstairs, the doorbell rings. When I answer it, I find a good-looking delivery man there with a large heavy package. He asks me to sign for it, and I ask if he wouldn't mind bringing it in for me, since it's so big. He says yes, and I ask him if he would bring it up to my bedroom. I get a suspicious look, but he agrees.

I follow him upstairs and tell him the truth. What's in the box has nothing to do with the bedroom, but I'm totally horny and I would love him to fuck me. I kiss him deeply and his response is all the answer I need. We strip quickly and get into bed. As he's kissing and touching and fingering me, he asks me if he can go down on me. His girlfriend doesn't let him and he loves doing it (hey . . . it's my fantasy!). I tell him I love that and he's welcome to, and I spread my legs for him.

Usually I come thinking about this stranger licking me to orgasm. Other times it's when he's deep inside me that I come. And some days I put my husband returning home early into the fantasy – and being touched and taken by both men gives me an explosive climax.

Name withheld, age 45
Heterosexual
Live-in relationship/marriage
Children
Some college
Writer
California, USA

I know what I really want now, before I just daydreamed. I want a tall man, with a thick cock, a great sense of humour, and the power to make things happen in his life. Before I wasn't sure what I wanted. My imaginary lover was just a dark figure with no real details. Now I fantasise about a famous man who finds my ass irritable as well as irresistible. We lock eyes in a crowded room and fireworks go off. He is over 6'4" and has blue eyes; he pushes my sexual safe buttons. We have a past life connection and we hump like rabbits. Sounds funny, but true.

Michelle, age 32
Heterosexual
Celibate
GCSE
Nanny
Location withheld, UK

I'm turned on by men with a nice smile or an accent. A gorgeous bottom always helps! I fantasise about some guy I fancy turning up on my doorstep and, before any words are spoken, he kisses me, rips off my clothes, and makes love to me right there in the hall, then the living room, the kitchen, the dining room, and finally the bedroom.

Natalie, age 40
Heterosexual
Live-in relationship/marriage
Children
Post-graduate coursework
Self-employed retail business/Property management
Arizona, USA

I fantasise about Tim McGraw (the country and western singer), having sex in public, sex with strangers, and sex with a younger man in his prime (since I'm in my prime right now). While I think about Tim McGraw often (and can direct my dreams in that way by listening to him before I go to sleep), lately I've been fantasising about my husband and trying new things with him. While we have amazing sex when we do, the frequency has lessened. He'd never had oral sex performed on him or anal sex until we got together. I try to think of new ways to please him in our real life, but my imagination and fantasies are a bit beyond him. I do enjoy minor bondage play, and he does get into that well. I feel that I'm a control freak in real life, and to be dominated is very exciting to me.

Here is my fantasy. I love Tim McGraw. He's such a sexy man with that black cowboy hat, perfectly coiffed facial hair, sultry come-and-get-me eyes and painted-on jeans. And, like a fine wine, he simply gets better with age – both physically and musically.

I listen to my Tim CDs all the time. 'Back When', while driving – his smooth voice calming potential road rage. 'Do You Want Fries With That', driving through McDonald's, absurdly praying he'll be the cashier. 'She's My Kind Of Rain', while masturbating in the bathtub – his manly, throaty purring mingling with vanilla bubbles, creating an irresistible sensory-stimulation spa.

I could listen to him all the time. 'Honey, could ya wash my shorts?' in that Louisiana-cum-Nashville accent. 'Sugar, we're out of toilet paper.' Glorious goose bumps.

Time for bed, radio on. Hubby is working late tonight. My CDs are parked in the car and I'm too lazy at the moment to get them. Ooooh! He's on the radio. I crawl beneath the sheets in my Tim nightshirt and lay my head upon my 250 thread-count Tim pillowcase, both recently acquired on eBay. The steady, repetitive chorus of 'Ticking Away' lulls me, comforts me and soothes me. I smell rain mingled with the night air while the mini-blinds bang against the window sill, keeping time with Tim's soulful crooning.

My fingertips feel my hardened nipples through Tim's glorious ironed-on portrait. A percussion of hair brushing the pillowcase's crinkly decal contributes lamely to the languor of the song. I feel for Tim, sitting in that bar, waiting for someone to enter and alleviate his loneliness. My eyelids are heavy. My pulse beats a rhythmic adagio as I drift off, my hand between my bare thighs.

A tickle upon my left shoulder stirs me. Did the dogs get in the house? I turn my head slowly, sighing. Tim's rigid image is slick beneath my sleep-sweaty hair. I hope I don't wrinkle him. I contemplate turning the pillowcase over. But then he'd suffocate. Another sigh. A noisy yawn. I blink my eyes. I blink them again. A black cowboy hat materialises on the pillow next to me, attached to Tim's head.

I lift the covers, praying for a body. There it is. Wow. Naked too. Hairy chest and all.

'How's it goin'?' That accent. I'm gonna have a coronary.

'Um, what are you doing here?' A falsetto voice, not mine.

'I got tired of sitting in the bar alone, so I grabbed a six-pack. It's in your fridge. Want one?' What? I'm having a multi-sensory delusion.

'No thanks. About the beer, I mean.'

'I'm gonna go snag me one then,' he drawls, rising from my bed. Hmmm. I guess his jeans aren't permanently attached. I wonder if baby oil would allow my 30-something-year-old ass to slide into my 20-something-year-old jeans.

'OK. Hurry back.' How lame. Tell him you're gonna miss him too.

With the full force of a hurricane I realise I am wearing his sexy persona on my boobs and crinkling his handsome face beneath my messy hair. I kiss the pillowcase and turn it over, hoping he can hold his breath a long time. I remove my shirt, folding it carefully and placing it gingerly on the floor. If my ultimate celebrity fantasy hallucination is naked, I should be too.

He slowly saunters back, taking a prolonged swig from the longneck bottle, his manhood swinging in the breeze, hat still on. Maybe it's sewn on. I should check. The hat, I mean. He climbs back into bed with me, placing the beer on the bedside table. I'm not going to worry about a coaster right now.

'So, what do you wanna do?' he asks, grinning behind a flirtatious wink of his magnificent eye. Sounds like a Cyclops. No, he has two eyes. Now that might be an interesting future fantasy: if Tim were missing one eye he might have an extra . . . My mind floods with a multitude of X-rated images, contortions, locations, props, extras. No, not extras. Well, maybe Chris Cagle. I'll put his CDs next to Tim's in my case for easy access.

My conscience hits me like a bolt of lightning from the tempest outside. I channel Benjamin Franklin. I lean over the foot of my bed, reaching for the dresser. Digging in a drawer

I produce a pair of my husband's boxer-briefs, waving them above my head, surrendering, scruples still intact.

'I'd feel better. They are clean.' He slips them on. Not as sexy as his jeans, but they'll do. Abruptly realising my own nakedness, I casually retrieve my nightshirt from the floor and yank it over my head.

'Nice shirt,' he observes. I smile, turning eleven shades of fuchsia. 'Want me to sign it for you?'

'Let me get a pen.' I leap out of bed, like a pad-less cat on a hot tin roof, and sprint down the hall in twelve seconds flat, unearth the Sharpie from the top of the refrigerator and race back. 'Here you go,' I pant, handing him the pen, cap removed for his convenience.

'Whoa. Slow down there.'

I lie on my back as he signs my boobs, his other hand on my belly holding his face still. I can't move until the ink dries. 'Thanks a lot,' I gush.

'Anytime.' Yeah, anytime I hallucinate you into my bed.

'Do you ever take your hat off?' I am nosy.

'Only in the shower.' Only? I am intrigued. I ask why. 'It's "The Cowboy in Me".' I should have known.

'You know I'm your number one fan.'

'Uh, please don't say that. It scares me in a Stephen King *Misery* sort of way.'

I giggle. 'Sorry, Mr McGraw.'

'Call me Tim.'

'Call me anytime. Oh, and "Please Remember Me".'

He chuckles. 'You're a funny one. Mind if I keep these?' He points at his luscious ass.

'Unless you want to moon the neighbours. I don't think my husband will miss them.'

He kisses me on the cheek, the tickle of his goatee titillating my every nerve. I'm never washing my face again. Then he left. Just left. Vanished. Disappeared. *Adios. Hasta la vista*, baby.

'I like it, I love it . . .' I had forgotten about the radio. Oh yeah, I'd love some more of him. I close my eyes, remembering the look in his eyes, the softness of his moustache on my skin, his fluid signature decorating my chest like icing on a cake. I check the ink. My nipples are so hard, I am afraid they'll poke his eyes out. I stroke my thigh, recalling his smell: a macho mixture of beer, testosterone and denim. Denim? I am soaked. My fingers slide across my clit. Randy Travis is on the radio now. I feel guilty masturbating to him. I sigh insufferably and crawl out of bed, adjusting the tuner on the radio. Tim, Tim, where are you? I need you.

Four stations later, the sweet strains of 'Let's Make Love' fly out of my radio and into my soul. Tim and Faith. Faith and Tim. The way it should be. All is right with the world now. I dance back into bed and close my eyes. My hand continues my extracurricular activities. I am happy. I am tired. I come. I sleep.

My husband climbing into bed at dawn awakens me. 'Did that come signed?'

3

Sex on the Edge

'Come to the edge, he said. They said, we are afraid. Come to the edge, he said. They came, he pushed them and they flew.'
                                                        – Guillaume Apollinaire

'Everything is sweetened by risk.'
                                – Alexander Smith

There's no doubt about it, women have become much more open-minded about their sexual interests and sexuality, even if they choose not to act upon it. There's now a lot more willing-ness to be experimental in the bedroom, and this naturally translates into the realm of sexual fantasy. As human beings, we love to explore, to imagine what can be found over the next horizon, what treasures can be uncovered, new sensations felt. We search for the same thrill we felt in that first tentative kiss with our lover, the thrill when we initially began to discover each other. We store these things in our memories and keep them close. But sometimes we dare to want more. Soon we find ourselves being drawn away from safe ground, moving further and further outwards until we finally come to the edge. Do we jump, or do we play at the brink?

This section is for those who have chosen to play at the brink – not quite taking that giant leap into empty space and possibly oblivion, but still defying the odds that the earth won't crumble beneath us and send us careening over the edge. We will explore fantasies that take a more daring turn away from the 'vanilla', that move into the shadows, although not into complete darkness. For some there is perhaps a fine line between what's considered 'on the edge' or in the 'danger zone' and, indeed, it's a highly subjective line, but for our purposes we'll reserve this section for those with a more adventurous streak. Here we have forbidden encounters, sex-toy play, outdoor sex and exhibitionism, threesomes, light bondage and S&M scenarios. We even take a dip into the realm of the fantastical, featuring encounters with the paranormal. It's all about adventure, a taste of the unknown ... It's all about playing on the edge.

Forbidden Fruit

Carolyn, age 44
Heterosexual
Live-in relationship/marriage
High School diploma
Writer
South Australia

I get turned on by men in uniform or in positions of power: politicians, police officers, soldiers, etc. As a result, I usually fantasise about a man in a position of power asking me to 'help' him in a sexual way. In my fantasy I'm at work in the tiny office I share with Mr X. We're talking about non-work things when he indicates that he wants me to come closer to where he's seated, next to his desk. I comply, and soon enough I'm sitting astride him. Somehow the door is locked and I can feel his appreciation of my actions tapping on my bum cheek. I reach down and release his penis, which is the most impressive one I've seen in terms of length and width. I shiver at the thought of having this organ invading my private territory – a shiver slightly of fear, but mostly of anticipation. I'm hardly a blushing virgin, I've been around, but this man, and his friend, are possibly more than I'd bargained on. Was there a promotion in his pants?

At that moment work was far from my thoughts. I climbed off Mr X's lap and knelt in front of the two of them, him and his dick, licking all the way. He held his hand out to me and made me stand, rubbing my clitoris with his hard penis the whole time. I couldn't control myself as I came, trying heedlessly to muffle my cries against his chest as I came, and came, and came. Mr X came with me, and, when the pleasure coursing through me slowed down and his mighty member spewed its last, I glanced at the carpet. Mrs Klemp was going to have a job of cleaning tonight, I said to myself, not caring at all. Mr X had his pleasure in hand and was rising to have another go, but this time we weren't going to go alone. I pushed him back to his executive chair and climbed onto his penis, riding him all the way to another bout of executive release as he sucked my nipples and I held onto his hard shoulders.

Alice, age 17
Heterosexual
Virgin
College student
Southeast England, UK

I'm turned on by loose natural clothing in beautiful colours. By contrast, I'm also turned on by crisp handsome businessmen (I always wonder what lies beneath their organised and anonymous exterior). Men in uniform, of course, particularly security guards and police officers are turn-ons. Heat, the sun, the sound of waves and running water, the tranquil sounds of nature in a forest or open countryside . . . I've recently taken a liking to guys who play guitar in a band. There's something really sexy about the way a guy pays so much attention to playing his guitar; it makes me wish I was his guitar and he was holding me against him and flicking my strings. The one thing that would definitely improve my sex life would be losing my virginity. Let me rephrase that: meeting the right person with whom I can feel totally comfortable having sex – 'mind sex', not just physical lust.

One of my favourite fantasies (an old one) involves a French teacher from secondary school a few years back. He is tall with dark curly hair and brown eyes that make you melt and has a deep voice with a sexy French lilt. It goes like this: I am in another lesson and the teacher asks me to get some exercise books from the staff room. When I enter the staff room it at first appears empty, but when I walk to the other side of the room where the books are I see that this French teacher, I'll call him Mr S, is sitting at a desk marking some papers. He looks up as I approach, and I say, 'Hi, Sir' to be friendly, hoping he hasn't noticed me blushing.

He looks back down at his papers, but I am aware that he's watching me closely as I bend down to look for the books. I find what I'm looking for and am about to turn around and head for the door when Mr S throws his pen down and says, 'Good homework, by the way. I've just finished marking it.' I mumble, 'Thanks', slightly embarrassed, as he gets up and moves towards me.

Am I imagining the playful twinkle in his eyes as he approaches? Probably. What would he see in an inexperienced schoolgirl anyway? The silence is intense as he looks me straight in the eye and gently traces his finger down my jaw. I think, 'OK, I am definitely not imagining this!' as he pulls me into him, and I can feel the whole length of his body, the heat radiating off him. My heartbeat goes mad as he bends down to kiss my neck, and I can feel the saliva he has left on me as he runs one hand through my hair while his other hand slides up my back.

Up to this point I'm too stunned to move, but I begin to respond by running my hands through his luscious dark curls and feeling his broad shoulders as they envelop me. The feel of his stubble brushing against my skin and the novelty of being so close that I can pick out each individual pore on his skin sends shivers down my spine. He likes this and smiles slightly as he slowly walks me backwards towards the table. I can feel his hard-on against my abdomen, and he slowly and deliberately grinds himself against my thigh as I'm pressed against the desk. By this point I am soaking wet and aching to feel him inside me, but reluctant to let him go further. I voice this reluctance, pointing out that another teacher could come in at any moment. 'I don't care,' he breathes in my ear. His hands move slowly as he begins to pull my tights down. When I make a move to escape, his strong arms grip me like a vice. His weight is pinning me down and I cannot move, my chest deliciously compressed under his. He becomes more frantic and in a couple of moments my school shirt is half ripped off me, my black lacy bra exposed. His tongue flickers over my breasts and down my stomach and he oh-so-gently kisses the skin, underneath which my womb is aching with anticipation. His hands move slowly between my legs and I pulsate beneath his long fingers as he moves them underneath my panties. I reach up and loosen his tie, undoing some of his shirt buttons. He can feel I'm ready, and unzips his trousers. Sometimes it is me who does this but I usually prefer the thought of him taking total dominance and overpowering me. When uncovered, his genitals are huge! At this point I feel very intimidated and he has to force my legs apart, all the while muttering in my ear in his lilting accent, coaxing me. Sometimes I give him oral first.

There are two different endings: the first one is that just as he is about to ease himself into me we hear voices outside the door and we both dive into a small room and block the door. There he proceeds to take my virginity and brings us both to bittersweet orgasm, but in near-total silence as the headmaster is now in the staff room drinking coffee! Or the second ending is along the lines of him making love to me over my newly marked homework on the desk. I then return to my lesson hot, sweaty and sore. My teacher tells me off for taking so long and my mates in the class all give me funny looks as I sit down and realise my shirt has a huge rip in it and I'm grinning like a Cheshire cat! I have several other fantasies involving my old sexy French teacher as he is very fantasy-worthy, but I could be here for days if I go through all of them!

Tami, age 36
Heterosexual
Live-in relationship/marriage
Children
Some college
Stay-at-home mom
Illinois, USA

When I was in eighth grade three really cute, popular boys from my class tricked me into going into a bedroom with them and then grabbed me and threw me down on the bed. They held me down and rubbed me all over. They didn't really go any further, but the feeling of being restrained and having all those hands all over me was something I will never forget. I don't know if that qualifies as the best sex I've ever had, but it probably left the biggest impression.

I have always loved to be dominated (but not hurt) by a very big strong guy. I love to fantasise about people who are in a position of trust – doctors, priests, nurses – forcing me to, or convincing me that I must, have sex with them. Sometimes I fantasise about being raped or gang-raped by large black men. They never hurt me and they are always very good about giving me pleasure. I have never been raped and I do not want to be raped for real. But in my fantasies it is all so good.

One of my favourite fantasies is about a trip to the gynie doctor (male or female, does not matter). I am in the stirrups and the doctor and nurse come in and proceed to examine my pussy, just looking and touching – no speculum! They decide I have a very unique pussy or a possible disease (it changes) and would like to observe me having an orgasm. They proceed to stimulate me to orgasm . . . the ways in which they do it always vary. Sometimes they make me stay completely still until I orgasm, which is very difficult. Sometimes they refuse to penetrate me until I orgasm, just letting me feel the head of a dildo against my pussy hole but not giving it all to me. Sometimes the doctor begs me to let him use his penis instead of the dildo even though he knows he could lose his licence, but he just has to be inside me. I always say yes!

Name withheld, age 37
Heterosexual
Live-in relationship/marriage
Children
Associate degree
Registered Nurse
Ohio, USA

The best sex I ever had was an encounter with a friend of a friend after I'd broken up with my boyfriend at the time. We were staying at a friend's house because we'd been drinking. We were both sleeping on the floor in the living room and had sex while my friends were in the other room asleep. It was a situation where we could have been caught at any time, and we weren't even 'dating' each other. But those facts made it feel forbidden and dirty.

Sometimes I wonder if I ran into someone who aroused me and the opportunity arose to act on it if I could really do it or not. I am married, though, and that holds me back. But as a fantasy it is very powerful. In my favourite fantasy, I have hot uncontrolled sex with an old boyfriend or stranger. At some point he puts me up on a table/dresser. My panties are around my ankles and his pants are around his ankles because we cannot wait to have each other. He can't keep his hands off me. It is a forbidden encounter.

Juliet, age 26
Heterosexual
Live-in relationship/marriage
Degree
University Administrator
East Anglia, UK

I've always had an obsession with sex. I masturbated frequently from the age of nine and still do. When I was fifteen I was watching a late-night TV show on the American porn industry, and there was a short clip on gay porn which really made me horny. I actually even now find it more appealing than lesbian scenes.

My job requires me to attend meetings, which of course are very boring. In some of these meetings there is an English lecturer who basically gets me wet when I see him. In my fantasy I can feel him eyeing me from across the room and catch some glimpses of him looking. After meeting some people I decide to go for a drink. I say that I will catch up after I tidy the room, but the lecturer doesn't leave. The next thing I know he's behind me touching my neck lightly with his fingers, then he starts to knead my breasts (which I like in real life). His hands find my zip, then work my trousers down to my knees. He inserts two fingers in my cunt, to which I let out the biggest moan, although still conscious that we're in a meeting room. Oddly, he doesn't say anything to me the whole time. I eventually turn around to face him and take my trousers off. I hitch myself onto a table and, with knees bent, I give him a full view of my cunt. I then have the best fuck and orgasm I've ever had.

Although I'm quite happy with my fantasy, I do feel that if the lecturer and I meet I would ask him to have sex with me.

Alexandra, age 27
Heterosexual
Single, very sexually active
College degree
Occupation unknown
London, UK

Where I grew up, it was one hundred per cent white middle class. The boys weren't interested in me for some reason. But I didn't really like them. I kept thinking, well, sex just isn't something that I really like. I thought it was boring. The white well-spoken boys bored me. Then I met a Brazilian guy who flipped my world upside down and I've never looked back! Now I adore sex, I'm such a sexual person. But I only like dark-skinned men, usually foreign.

I have so many fantasies, but my favourite is being approached by a sixteen-year-old teenage boy, black, usually Caribbean. He hits on me, and I laugh in his face because he doesn't realise how old I am (I look young). When I tell him that I'm 27, he looks shocked, then smiles. He's tall, over six feet, with beautiful cheekbones, skin, teeth and gorgeous eyes, which have a slightly cruel/bad boy look to them. We flirt and I tell him he has no chance with me. He tells me that I'll never have it as good as I would with him. I keep laughing at him, because he's so cocky and arrogant (as most teenage boys are!). But I can see something in him, the way he walks, talks, holds himself, the way he looks at me. He's not a virgin and he's been with women who have told him that, yes, he's as fine as he thinks he is. My curiosity gets the better of me and I give him my number. His testosterone is like a heat shimmer around him. He's too hot, too young, too fine . . .

He calls me later that week and tells me (not asks me) he's coming over. He turns up just after I've got back from work. I'm in a work skirt suit and heels and I know I look good. The skirt makes my butt look curvy and big, and my waist look tiny. He's wearing a T-shirt and I can see his ripped muscular arms and pecs. His baggy jeans hang off his hips, showing just a taster of flesh on his stomach. As he stands behind me while I make him a drink, I can feel his body heat and he smells so good. He puts his hands around my waist and I arch my back and push my ass towards him. He slides his hands down to my ass and whispers in my ear that I'm the finest white woman he's seen. I turn around and we kiss. He bites my lip, teasing me. I pull his T-shirt over his head. His body is *amazing*. I can't tell you what muscles covered in black skin do to me. He even has some tattoos covering his biceps. I just want to bite him, eat him all up. I spend minutes just smoothing my hands over his body, as he bites my neck and shoulders … You know what? It's not even about the sex. It's about his body and how good it looks and feels to touch and how salty and warm his skin is. I'm obsessed by bodies like this. It's his dark skin against my lightness. It's his youth, how perfect he is. I know boys like this, and all I do is stare at them. Stare so much. I can't have them, so I get what I need from staring.

S, age 22
Heterosexual
Steady relationship/not live-in
Bachelor's degree
Writer
Dublin, Ireland

I like the idea of forbidden sex … and I get really turned on by guys with plump sexy lips. I used to have a boyfriend with these amazing bedroom eyes and full lips! He was so beautiful in a sort of feminine-model way, but he was also really masculine; he really did it for me! I like spontaneous sex. I love to be able to chat to a guy for hours on end and really connect on a mental level first; it makes the sex so much better. I like cheeky boys who know how to tease endlessly without being too mean. Big willies also, it goes without saying. The thought of being dominated (like thrown over the edge of a couch or tied up) is quite sexy. I also like the idea of being the innocent schoolgirl type in a short skirt being corrupted by the bad man! I think this was my sexually repressed Catholic upbringing.

Imagine this ... you have been carved into this perfect young lady. All-girls' convent, university education ... sex was never really discussed in your household. You learned all you know from poring through magazines and books, and reading about blow jobs and sex in aeroplanes. Now imagine coming to maturity and wanting to rebel against it, yet have it in every way possible – in your mind, body and soul. To completely surrender to it.

In my fantasy I am wearing a very short skirt. It's a school skirt pleated and high on my thighs, which in the fantasy are long, slim and tanned. Underneath I am wearing white lacy pants, which make me feel sexy and naughty, stockings up to my knees, and a school shirt. I am the ultimate juxtapose: naughty, hungry and dirty on the inside; sweet, happy and innocent on the outside.

I am in school that day, aged about seventeen, and wearing what I described above. The young training teacher tells me he needs to keep me behind. 'I want to see you after class, young lady,' he says good-naturedly, winking. In his mid-20s and fresh out of college, he's tall and good-looking with lovely masculine hands, piercing eyes that look right into you, and a cheeky grin. Every girl in the class has a crush on him. After everyone leaves, I'm sitting at my desk waiting for him to come and talk to me. He shuffles his papers and, when he's sure everyone has gone, approaches me to ask why I haven't done my homework. Looking up at him from my chair, I reply that I just didn't want to. He is wearing a white shirt and a tie, and he loosens it a bit and sits down beside me quietly and puts his hand on my leg, which is now tensing at his touch, sending lightning blots through my whole body. Our eyes meet – he looks me up and down lustily and I know what's going through his mind. He then gets up and closes the blinds and locks the classroom door. He sits back down and tells me I have been a bad girl and I need to learn my lesson. He then runs his hands right up my thigh to my lacy pants; he pulls them aside with his fingers and pushes his hands roughly into me. I suck my breath in, biting my lip, and he pushes them in deeper. He then kisses me gently and grabs my hand, putting it on his crotch where I can feel his hard cock through his trousers. He then tells me to get up on the desk. I do that and he tells me, 'No, I want you to kneel on the desk.' So I do what he says, getting on the desk on my hands and knees like a cat, my bum in the air. I am tense for a moment, wondering what he will do next. He rubs me again, sending volts of electricity up my spine. He takes my pants and he pulls them down to my knees. Then he pulls up my skirt, spreading my legs wider apart. He puts his head under my skirt and licks me with his strong tongue, gasping as he does. My head is arched back and I'm shivering. He then undoes his button and takes out his cock in his hand, rubbing it openly. I turn around and sit on the desk, opening my legs and undoing my shirt. He has a look of ecstasy in his eyes as he massages his dick. He puts his free hand up my skirt once more and I throw my shirt on the floor. Then I undo my bra, and sit back on the desk. He gives me a dirty look and comes over to me, kissing my breasts for a minute, then kissing my face frantically. He pushes my head down, forcing me to suck him until he is rock hard and moaning. He pulls up my head and gets me to turn around once more. He probes his cock against me and we both let out a gasp. Then quickly he enters me, forcefully. He grabs my hair and pulls on it, my neck back, my spine arched as he pumps harder and faster . . .

And it pretty much ends there I'm afraid. Hopefully teachers like this will never be employed in real life!

Kele, age 21
Heterosexual
Celibate
University degree
Student
Western Cape, South Africa

I'm turned on by fantasies about ex-boyfriends, where the relationship has ended dismally, and they're fingering me to orgasm. In my fantasy he stands above me and torments me until I give in. He doesn't tease, he doesn't listen to my pleas. He just forces his hands and makes me come so hard I think I'll fall apart. Just when it's subsiding, he starts again and I'm rocking with the sensation. I hate him. I hate the way he hurt me. I hate that no one has made me feel like he has in three years. I hate this on-off thing we keep having. I hate that when I see him my whole body goes into shock again. I hate the small town we live in where I bump into him almost daily, at the library, in the supermarket. I hate that he rejected me before. I hate that I'm loving his smell, his feel, his taste so much. I can't stand him but I can't say no.

We met in the club tonight, and I knew it was time to leave. I had to walk past him to get out and, as I did so, he greeted me casually. I barely looked at him because his eyes burned into me. But I had to look back; is this really him? He smiled in that knowing way, his latest girlfriend on his arm, grinning prettily (bitch!). I swore I would never be alone with him. When I came out of the toilet, he pushed me into the cubicle hastily. And before I knew it I had sunk again. His lips, oh God, that man makes my head spin every time he kisses me. My legs open of their own accord. And he whispers, 'I knew you couldn't resist me. Since that first day, I know you've wanted this.' I can't even deny it, I've been craving him for so long. I know he doesn't love me. I know it will never be anything more, but, God, I need this. It's been three years since he touched me and nobody can even come close. I've been celibate for two years now, can't even make myself come without thinking about him. And now he's here, and it feels so good, but I have to stop. 'This isn't right. You can't just show up and fuck me up all over again, Nkuli.'

'I'm not asking,' he answers as his hands pull up my skirt roughly. I'm bending over the toilet, and he's behind me and he's so rough it almost hurts; it's so good. I feel his jarring inside me from behind with one hand over my clitoris. Oh, God, I need this, but I must stop this. 'Come on, just let go.' I wish he wasn't right. What choice do I have, I can feel it coming. And I'm a screamer, but he puts his free hand against my mouth to contain the sound. Oh shit, this is so good …

Shanna, age 18
Heterosexual
Virgin
College Student
Singapore

In my favourite fantasy, a guy is sitting in the back of his chauffeured car (the windows are tinted) waiting for his seventeen-year-old niece. She gets in the car unsuspectingly. They get into foreplay and her uncle suckles her virgin twat. He laps up her juices and plays around her labia with his tongue. (Keep in mind the girl is wearing her school uniform.) She moans. They rock the limousine, and shouts of pleasure and their lascivious moans can be heard outside the car.

The chauffeur gets off on their muffled sex cries, and passers-by are intrigued.

Unearthly Pleasures

Sheila, age 34
Heterosexual
Steady relationship, not live-in
High School diploma
Occupation unknown
Ohio, USA

I liked being in control of sexual situations when I first learned about sex. Experience has led me to become a female dominant. In the relationship I have now it is vanilla D/s. In the past I have been a switch (someone who can be either the dominant or submissive with their partner). My experience with women has mainly been through BDSM, kissing, touching and use of toys and props with them, but I have yet to have a full-on female experience. If the right woman came along I very well could give it try, I think. The lesbian curiosity is one that I would like to explore because I believe it would be so different being with someone who knows in her own way what I would like, could understand my thoughts and feelings better. What keeps it from happening, not really searching for it, is that I know that relationships are relationships; no matter your sexual orientation, each group has its own problems. So I think, why trade the problems that I am used to for a different set? Besides, I do love men a hell of a lot and I damned sure enjoy being dominant over the man in my life.

Though I am dominant, the best sex came when I was in a

submissive role. I was with a man and we were doing age-play role-playing, dad/daughter scene. He had a way of making me feel very young even though he was not much older than me. I was pleasing 'daddy' orally, trying to make up for being a very bad girl, when the man's real-life brother walked in on us. OMG! Embarrassment and shock at getting caught in the exposed position I was in were only a few of the feelings going through me, not to mention I was extremely horny, too! A look, a few words between the dominant 'daddy' and me, and we invited the brother to join us. This night became my first, and so far only, experience with a threesome. Still makes me drip thinking about it. And yes, the brother stepped in to the role of 'uncle' to the dad/daughter scene.

Erotica and romantic erotica are my first reading choices when possible, followed by paranormal romances and so on. When it comes to fantasy, the themes I go to often are paranormal, like vampires (as victim or as the vamp) and werewolves, BDSM, inanimate objects (for example, statues), and some taboo subjects such as rape and incest. Some fantasies have force to mild violence. What holds me back from living out my fantasies? Vampire fantasy is hard to complete, don't you think? Role-playing is as close as I get to that one, and it's freaking hot when I play that role, too. Finding a statue that can fill the role of my latest fantasy isn't easy. And rape is not anything I want to have happen to me or anyone else.

Recently the fantasy that gets me going is sex with a statue. It plays out this way: I'm a woman who is at an art auction. I'm exploring the items up for bid and come across a wonderfully aroused sculpted male statue, one that to my mind puts the statue of David to shame. Though I'm there with my mind set on a certain painting, something about the statue calls to me and I set out to win it, and do. The statue is delivered. Alone with it at last, I can't stop touching it. The more I touch it the more aroused I become and I figure out a way to impale myself on its sculpted cock and come.

The only real variance in the above fantasy is that sometimes the statue will come to life while I'm riding it and other times not.

Cecilia, age 40
Bisexual
No children
Live-in relationship/marriage and steady relationships, not live-in
Master's degree
Writer
Massachusetts, USA

I discovered I could masturbate to orgasm when I was about five years old. Even then, images of bondage and power/domination turned me on – Catwoman and Batman on the old *Batman* TV show, the episode of *Star Trek* with the slave people . . . I like to fantasise about men on men, bondage, role-playing, cock worship, large cocks and what to do with them, domination, gay love, and beautiful young men. There are lots more but in the past six to eight months those are the top themes.

In my fantasy I'm a young prince whose father is involved in a huge power struggle. The scenario can vary from the family being modern crime lords, to medieval settings with magic and spells. My safety has been entrusted to an older man whom I gradually fall in love (or at least lust) with, but when my father discovers that this man is actually a traitor working for our enemies he is forced to flee, taking me with him. Sometimes I start out as a hostage, sometimes I have secretly been helping him all along to bring my father down. Either way, we end up in a deeply sexual relationship, fuelled by the tension.

The scenario climaxes when my father catches up to us at last – we know he's spying on us but hasn't yet made his move, and, to protect me, my lover enacts a scene in which he 'rapes' me, to make it look to my father like I've been his captive, his slave all along, when in truth it is our goodbye.

Cynthia, age 31
Bisexual
Single, moderately sexually active
No children
Master's degree
Residence Hall Director
Ohio, USA

I'm turned on by sexual tension, especially when I can't act on it. But flirting with the person and playing with fire is always fun. I'm a little less caught up on hearts and flowers and champagne. Romance is wonderful, but I'm also attracted to raw sexuality, being sexually satisfied. When I was younger, I was more worried about pleasing my partner than myself.

Lately, I've fantasised about having sex with a very alpha male, one who is almost controlling. I have a favourite fantasy about being taken (literally kidnapped) by a man who is superhuman in some way (vampire, werewolf, wizard, etc.). He takes me to his home, which is somewhere secluded, to be used as his sexual plaything. Sometimes he locks me in a little cage, sometimes he chains me to his bed, and other times he uses some sort of magical power on me in order to bend me to his will. He likes to tease me. He pulls my ass to the edge of the bed and then ties my legs open so they are completely stretched out. That way he has access to my ass and my pussy. The man only wants me as a sexual servant but eventually develops feelings for me. While I enjoy having sex with him, I am angry with him for holding me captive. The fantasy usually ends with me tying him up and leaving him unsatisfied as I walk out.

Name withheld, age 46
Heterosexual
Live-in relationship/marriage
Bachelor's degree
Writer
Wisconsin, USA

When I was young I thought Robert Plant of Led Zeppelin (when he was in his early 20s) was beautiful. Of course, I was very young and inexperienced (thanks to a very protective dad), and so my mind couldn't grasp anything beyond hugging and kissing. Now I'm turned on by nude Greek statues, the kind found in museums. You have these healthy, trim gods doing their thing – chasing nymphs or what have you. The sculptors should have shown these statues masturbating or getting their cocks licked, because all that beauty is otherwise going to waste. Walking through a major art museum is better than a porn movie any time!

My fantasies mostly revolve around the theme of being put in a situation where I can't really be held responsible for my actions. For example, my engaging in the act is the lesser of two evils. (It's like you have a choice: either the guy performs cunnilingus on you and your friend, or you have to act as maid for the 3-storey, 115-room whorehouse. And, may I add, you have no help in cleaning the house. It's room after room of scrubbing toilets, wiping down shower walls, and cleaning someone's hairs out the sink. I hate picking hairs out of the sink!)

Well, my actual fantasies are much more concrete than that.

This is to say, I don't fantasise about a guy sticking his prick up my ass because I know from experience that, unless the guy knows what he's doing, the act hurts like hell. I don't fantasise about having two guys lick me at the same time because I know someone is going to get pissed off at somebody else. Someone is going to feel left out. And the United States is still largely heterosexual, so it's damn unlikely that two het males are going to feel comfortable about rubbing against each other (and I'm sure if you have two males to one woman, one of the males is bound to accidentally touch the other male, and then you have two males ready to fight because someone feels that his masculinity is being challenged. Every het male I've talked with regarding multiple partners expressed indignation about touching another naked male).

OK, here goes (blush). I'm on my hands and knees, being slow-fucked by two witches. I don't mean they're fucking me slowly. I mean the auburn-haired witch who kneels behind me has his hands on my hips, and he pushes his huge dick in me real fast, and then he pulls out really slow, so that I feel every morsel of delicious friction as he withdraws his cock. He never completely withdraws. He's just in real hard and real fast, and out real tender and slow as though he knows how to let his cock linger on the edge of my pussy. If I could, I would scream, but the 6' 4" black-haired, blue-eyed babe who kneels before me, well, he looks even better without any clothes. He's cut, with the six-pack and the guns. He doesn't look like a high priest in one of the most whispered-about covens in the region. He looks like a weightlifter from one of those expensive California gyms. This ain't California, though, and he wears nothing but a blue tattoo of the Horns of Isis on his right shoulder and a silver pentagram with an amethyst as its centrepiece around his throat.

The auburn witch halts, leans into me a little, and begins to finger my clit. The more the auburn pagan pinches the lips of my pussy and squeezes my clit between his index and third finger, the harder I suck the black witch. God in Heaven, he tastes so creamy and smooth – like sweet yogurt when you add a tiny bit of salt. He strokes my hair and shifts his hips a little. Suddenly he pushes me backwards and the auburn one pulls at my shoulders until I'm flat on my back. I stare at the ceiling – a beautiful painting that depicts every known goddess exposing her swollen cunt to the hungry mouth of a god with a rig not to be believed. Auburn brings his face close to mine so that I see his long straight lashes, which are rather pale when compared to the sensual reds and soft browns of his hair. He pins my wrists to the dirt floor and shoves his tongue inside my mouth. The high priest thrusts my legs apart, revealing my cunt which makes a wet smacking sound as the lips of my vulva open a little. Oh goddamn! Resting his weight on his elbow and knees, the black priest uses one of his hands to guide himself inside me. I gasp for air as his tremendous-sized dick tears its way through my walls. I scream from a good pain because I need to be fucked raw. I am two weeks away from my bleeding, and I have become mad, mindless and chaotic in my need to have a dick inside me and my clit licked and nibbled. My arms snake around his shoulders, my legs embrace his hips. During the two weeks prior to my period, I can think of nothing except making the horniness go away. His hips guide mine into a rhythmic sway. His razor stubble rakes my face. He's deep inside me, nourishing me in this crumbling, forgotten church with its busted-out windows and the occasional crow flapping through the mouldy air. Vaguely, I think if we're caught bare-assed and screwing inside an abandoned church, then who is going to bail our asses out of jail? Actually, I'm thinking who is going to bail *my* ass out of jail? Like many witches, Black Hair is middle-to-upper class, well-educated, and a phone call away from a lawyer who probably plays golf with the district attorney every Sunday. Me? I'll be lucky if I land a cell *above* the ground. 'Don't worry about it,' he lifts himself on his elbows but he doesn't stop fucking me. He has the hard, angular features of the Norwegians, but the full, pouting lips of the Swedes. When he smiles, his face softens. 'I'm a witch, remember?' Sometimes, balling a witch can get a little creepy because he can be eerily telepathic. For now, though, his fucking feels too good for me to argue with him.

Toy Stories

Astrid, age 58
Heterosexual
Live-in relationship/marriage
Children
PhD
Writer
Vienna, Austria

My fantasy is written as a story. The only time my mother spoke to me about sex was when I was fifteen. It was an effort to demystify the contents of my womb with the help of illustrations in my zoology book. I do not have memories of ever having been told to keep my fingers out of 'there', although I do recall how I told my two-year-old daughter that one did not do 'that' with people around. And although I cottoned on later to what he was getting at, I'm sure that my mother, one of those women who eventually gets everything right, never wanted to go into the reasons for Mick Jagger singing, 'I can't get no satisfaction'. Or maybe she knew that in the end it was not satisfaction that was the game's name.

All these jumbled thoughts played through my mind as I waited for my plane for New York and my menopause to strike. My ovaries were having what I thought was their final fling, yet I still wondered why I was suddenly in such a state of enduring arousal. I told my muse, but his reaction did not solve the problem, if problem there was.

'Are you still horny?' he asked me before I left.

'I think I'll be horny for ever.'

'Music,' he said.

Yes, my muse is a man. Who else could coax the unspeakable from within my core to my breast and down the length of my arms to my right hand, through my fingers, the pen, the keys, to the page? Music, yes. But he wasn't around and it wasn't really about him. It was about me.

More and more I wanted to explore. I would have dreams of dancing naked in a roomful of dildos. There were black ones and red ones, purple, yellow; there were big ones and curved ones, ones with glitter and with little appendices; what they all had in common were smiles on their dickheads. I wanted books on my shelves about cock, clit and cunt, but I wanted nice covers.

Just like Hook's Peter Pan before he could fly, I'd missed the 60s. But it wasn't too late to play with the forbidden. Four-letter words. Fuck was one I had started to say aloud, but only when swearing; then there was cock as in peak, cunt as in hunt, clit as in split. And oh so much more in the name of love. I wanted to play with anal and bang, blow, buns and bush, butt, come and slit. I wanted oils and creams, candles and lubes. In an orgy of the senses I wanted to drown. I wanted to learn how to masturbate, do a course, start from scratch. I didn't want mail order. I wanted someone to take me in hand. A shop. Friendly staff. I had questions to ask.

I'd sent an email from the town of Calvin in Switzerland

where I lived. No sex shops in the city? One. Two. Maybe more tucked away in the red-light area behind the station. I scuttled in once for a look and scuttled out again with my clandestine purchase of pink pleasure balls, a present to me on my 52nd birthday. My mother's day gift was the trip to New York and a tube to the lower east side. Babes in Toyland. The musical. No way.

My heart was beating as I pushed open the door. Over eithteen. You betcha. So why did I feel nervous? Wow! It was gorgeous. So was she. Like the girl next door. I've always had a soft spot for tomboyish redheads. From my Pippy Longstocking days, I guess. At the threshold I let slip the coat of being a wife, a mother, from my shoulders. I only had that afternoon in the store. It was now or never. I had to do the necessary research. I was a writer, a lover, and I was going to learn how to write erotica. My head spun. It was gorgeous, I felt dizzily free.

'So you made it?' she said. 'Come. Put your bag down and I'll show you around.'

'Do you have the same size, but without the vanilla taste?' The words floated across from a table of dildos. A voluptuous black woman wistfully stroked a large curved purple number and I stared as if in a trance.

'Do you want to start with the dildos?' the redhead said.

I put my bag down, shook my head. It was spinning. Then I blurted, 'I don't know what I want. This is my first time. Can you show me ... the Hitachi wand?'

The redhead raised one eyebrow and then she smiled. She was gentle and pretty. Freckles sprinkled her nose. She picked up the biggest vibrator I had ever seen. Now this wasn't difficult since I'd only seen the mail-order ones intended for easing pain in the neck region. I could never get that 'wand' inside me. Then I realised that was perhaps not the main intention. The redhead turned it on.

'Do you have something a little more ... discreet? In size and in sound?'

She showed me a tiny finger cap. 'It comes with its own little purse to slip on a belt.'

I could just see myself travelling with my bumbag and the mini-vibe purse. 'Is it any good?'

She turned it on. It gave a low buzz. 'I need something a little more powerful myself,' she confided.

'Looks fine to me,' I said. 'I'm just a beginner. I'll take the purple one.' Purple seemed to fit my mood perfectly.

'There are books there. A wonderful one called simply *Clit*.'

'I was looking for *The Best of*,' I said. 'I can't get those in Geneva.'

'There are no sex shops?'

'Not like this. I bought some pink balls though. They were the only things discreet enough. It was a shop in the middle of town,' I added hastily.

'And how are they?'

'The balls?'

The redhead nodded.

'I tried them once. I didn't dare bring them.'

'X-rays at the airport,' she said and shook her head.

'Oh, my God. Wearing the balls and then having them ding as you go through the controls.' I started to giggle.

The redhead giggled with me. 'There's worse,' she said. 'Wear a harness to JFK and see where that gets you.'

'I'm not that far yet,' I said.

She smiled and gave me a postcard. 'There's a masturbation marathon this Sunday. You're welcome to come.'

I took the card. A 40s-type playmate, who reminded me of my mother, sat atop a Hitachi wand, stroking her cheek with a daisy. Masturbate-A-Thon. 'I'd love to,' I said. 'But I fly out that night. I'm here for a meeting. Work.'

The redhead nodded. 'Another time then.'

'I'll just have a look at the books before I go.' I didn't want to leave, but I had to. I was awaited in my hotel by the Empire State Building. There was no pocket of time for me to come back. I bought three anthologies and the purple finger fiddler. It was a start. When the mind loosens the vagina luxuriates.

Back in Geneva the Earth Mother was calling. I had to nurture and care for and hold those I loved. But I would fantasise, and my cunt would drip with Tahitian pearls as my muse fondled my puckering butthole with creamy fresh butter, his fingers slipping so gently, easing, stroking and poking, making way for his cock so eager to sink home, and thrusting me beyond space and time.

Then came the eleventh day of September. I emailed the redhead. She said she was safe.

I slept in chunks of three or four hours. I did not have headaches, but the Earth Mother in me had to learn once again as I tried to pretend I was still this side of bruised. And so I curled up like the child I once was, hiding my hands between my thighs, seeking safety and comfort in that foetal position. It was then that my fingers began their own life and traced gently to dip to my moist inner reaches, and I rubbed and I rubbed until I found sleep.

Josie, age 36
Bisexual
Live-in relationship/marriage
Children
Master's degree (PhD candidate)
Computer programmer/Website designer/Writer
Wales, UK

I've always had a vivid imagination but now I have more ideas to work with. I've seen more and done more, so a lot of my fantasies are based on memories of good times rather than plans for the future. But I still do fantasise about things I've never done. I think that I fantasise a lot more about men now that I'm comfortable with being a lesbian. This sounds strange, but when I was a teen, I was quite militant about lesbianism as I felt I had to continually prove that I was really a dyke and not going through a phase. This was mainly because people kept telling me I was too pretty to be a lesbian and crap like that, so being turned on by a man or men in general made me feel guilty. It doesn't bother me any more now – I know that my fantasies are my own and not for anyone else's judgement. Just because I fantasise about sex with men doesn't mean I have to move one in with me and cook his dinner, wash his dirty pants, and listen to him gobbing on about football and cars, ewk.

I fantasise a lot of scenarios, with the lead up to having sex, the situation, build-up, romantic stuff. There used to be a lot of touching and kissing but very little else in my fantasy; usually they involved a particular person, e.g. a film star (female). This went on for years after I became sexually active, so it wasn't about not knowing what to do. Lately, since my late 20s I'd say, my fantasies have been much more graphic. Hang the build-up, I just want the sex! They involve strangers mainly (feels less guilty than thinking about friends), male and female, both at once, group orgies. I often still have the build-up ones too. Some recurring themes are that I pick up a prostitute (either while I'm pretending to be a man), or I pick up a butch dykey type and I play the high-class whore – very unrealistic as my prostitutes are usually healthy and intelligent and I take them out to dinner and woo them beforehand. I'm rich and pay for everything, of course.

Another theme is the deflowering of a virgin – an older teen shy boy, where I teach him what to do, and there's a similar one with a girl, where I get her to strap on a dildo and show her the ropes there as well. A lot of it is about control. I'm calling the shots, but at the end I'm on my back totally out of control.

Women in uniform appear quite a bit; often I'm in prison and there's a sexy guard who knows how to use her truncheon, so there's power play too. I'm not always in control. Uniforms, muscled women (body-builders, martial arts, etc., but not overly muscled), tattoos, women in men's suits – this makes me sound butch-obsessed, but I'm also turned on by stockings/suspenders, make-up, revealing dresses, glam. I swing both ways in that I'm turned on by wearing this stuff and by others wearing it as well. I also like to see men in drag. I'm such a perv!

I never thought I would, but I have a Pavlovian reaction to the sight of a strap-on dildo. Initially I thought they were hilarious and couldn't get turned on by them, but, after about ten years of using one, the association with pleasure overrides how ridiculous it looks. I got a leather jacket when I was nineteen, and have since been very turned on by leather clothes. I especially like feminine women wearing leather, for instance a basque. I love burlesque on men and women. I like contradictions, butch and femme clothes in a mix, such as wearing stockings with kick-ass boots, gender fuck stuff. I think that's why I like drag queens and drag kings.

I love to strap on a dildo and fuck a woman, and I also love to be fucked in the same way. I like a slow build-up, I'm quite tight at first and need to get worked up before I can enjoy the penetration. But then once I'm going at it, it's the best thing ever. That's why I can't get going with men because, by the time I'm warmed up, they're already finished. Unless it's a whole rugby team, lol.

I have enough material for a feature film-length fantasy. I've deliberately written it quite matter-of-factly as I can't stand purple prose. Sometimes I get all the way through this fantasy on insomnia nights; sometimes I skip to the chase or dwell on particular scenes. In my fantasy I'm a wealthy businesswoman; I've made a killing on the internet, selling sexy underwear and sex toys. I've decided to open a club in LA or San Francisco, and have to travel there to scout out the place. I contact an escort agency to set me up with someone who can act as my guide. I select the guide I want based on photos (she's young, butch dykey, spiky hair, etc., a bit like Shane from *The L Word* but not so skinny, more muscled), and get to know her via email before I go. The trip is due to be a month long, and I pack one case full of business suits plus another of stock: sexy clothes and my own brand of sex toys.

At the airport my cases are opened and the (female) guards see the contents. I'm taken to a private room for a stripsearch by two guards. Predictably, they are both gorgeously butch. I flirt with them while they're searching and they flirt back. Then they ask me about the toys in my case and I demonstrate to them. They watch while I masturbate, then use the toys on me and on each other. Two hours later I manage to catch my flight.

It's a long flight and I try to sleep for some of the way. However, I can't sleep as I'm uncomfortable in the seats, so I call an air hostess. She's very feminine and sexy and gives me the come-on look. I tell her I can't sleep and she says that the first-class compartment is empty – I can use that if I like, and she joins me there. We kiss and she says it's her first time with another woman. She wants me to fuck her, which I do.

I get to LA and I'm met by my escort, who is even sexier in person than in her photos. She takes me to my hotel and shows me around, then leaves me to sleep. She is friendly and I flirt with her, but she is quite cool and professional with me and doesn't flirt back. The next day we go through my plans. I want her to show me around the various clubs, shops and sex shows in town, and introduce me to some people. She says we'll start with a lap-dancing club.

We go to the club and watch some dancing on stage, then my escort asks if I want to get a dance from a girl. I say yes, and ask if she's going to get one too. She says she won't. We go to an area behind the stage and I sit there while this scantily clad girl writhes all over me. Meanwhile, my escort leans against the wall watching us and smiling slightly. At first I'm disconcerted and a bit embarrassed that she's watching, but I forget she's there and enjoy what the girl is doing. Every club we go to things like this happen. The escort acts as my protection, so that I can go and do anything I want and she'll stay on guard and stay sober, but she always watches. I feel her eyes on me when I'm having sex with prostitutes at the back of a club, or when I'm dragged up onstage by a stripper. Anything that happens, the escort is there.

Several times I make a move on the escort but she gives me the brush-off. She says she doesn't get involved with her clients. She stays professional with me and never lets me get intimate with her, although she sees me in various states of sexual excitement, inebriation and undress. I am deliberately provocative knowing that she's watching. I get sleazy and dirty. Eventually I stop enjoying the sex with other people, because I want her so much. I'll be lying there letting someone fuck me and I spend the whole time making eye contact with the escort while she stands in the corner of the room with her arms folded.

The month passes in a haze and it's my last night there. I've established some business contacts and have agreed on a premises; it's all going smoothly. I tell my escort that I won't need her services any more as I'm going home the next day. I decide that I'll stay in the hotel that night. We say goodbye and I settle up her fee. But that night I can't sleep and I decide to just go out for one last time. I head to one of the clubs my escort has taken me to before. I'm enjoying the show when out of the corner of my eye I spot her: my escort! She hasn't seen me because she's engrossed in flirting with this femmy woman whom I recognise as someone I had sex with while I was last here. They leave together and I follow them.

They go to an alley behind the club, and I hide behind some bins to watch them have sex. I am so turned on now, because in all this time that she has been watching me do things like this I've never seen her being anything but aloof and cool. I had assumed she was celibate or didn't like sex. Now she's losing it with this woman and I'm itching to join in. But I don't. Something stops me from approaching her, I feel anxious that there must be something about me that turned her off. After they've finished, they begin to walk back to the club and the other woman goes on ahead while the escort lingers. I have to squeeze behind the bins to hide, but I knock one of them over. She turns around and sees me.

The escort is angry that I've followed her and she shouts at me. I shout back, saying I had thought in all this time she had high ideals and that's why she didn't want to fuck me but she's just a slut after all. She gets more angry and we start to fight and, as we're struggling, she kisses me. Then she breaks down and says that it wasn't that she didn't want me, but that she wanted me too much. She knew if she allowed herself to feel for me then she wouldn't be able to bear it when it was time for me to go back home.

We go back to the hotel and we have the most amazing sex that lasts all night. I unpack my case of toys and we use everything several times – she straps it on for me and fucks me senseless. It's the best sex ever. In the morning, of course, I will have to go home, but I don't usually get to that part. In the fantasy the night never ends.

Pamela, age 51
Heterosexual
Live-in relationship/marriage
Children
Some college
Freelance Writer/Editor
Iowa, USA

I grew up with all of my uncles' and dad's friends around, mostly musicians and race car drivers. When I was about thirteen, I became enamoured with my dad's friend who wore silk shirts and a gold watch. The sleeves were always unbuttoned and the cuffs rolled up twice. He always left a couple of buttons undone, and he had a very hairy chest. Once I asked him if I could feel his shirt and he let me. To this day I cannot resist that look. I used to encourage my husband to dress like that. Touching his chest and feeling his muscles was one of my biggest turn-ons. I also love men with long hair. I married at sixteen, and, yes, he is an older man, six years older, in fact. Experienced older men still turn me on big time. I still love silk on both men and women, and long hair really gets to me. Handcuffs and men's aftershave – certain kinds – trigger memories that really get me hot.

When I first started fantasising, I didn't really touch myself. Well, I did, but not to orgasm, just more to get turned on. It wasn't until I was sixteen and married and had an orgasm that I began wanting to orgasm when fantasising. Now that I'm more mature, I have a toy-box full of toys and I actually orgasm every time. I also have an online dominant lover who helps with that. The one thing holding me back is the fact that my husband does not understand my submissive needs and it would hurt him if I went elsewhere to a real dom. He is very vanilla and no matter how I try to explain it, he just doesn't get it. I have never kept secrets from my husband and he knows I have an online dominant.

Some of my fantasies revolve around memories, but go further than the actual happenings. My favourite fantasy takes place in the bathtub. Master is bathing me and he uses the massage head on my clit, making me orgasm over and over. Here's a little story I wrote to my dom about my favourite fantasy. I call it *An Email to My Lover*:

Hello Darlin'...

I am missing You so bad. I wrote this today after my shower. I so wanted You there with me. You know how much I hate playing alone. I hate that You had to work today. Imagine the insensitivity of a company that thinks You need to actually work for the money they pay You! LOL.

As I slipped into the warm water I could feel You there with me ... smell the soft lilac scent of the bath salts I used ... feel the touch of Your hands ... hear Your soft voice whispering to me ...

Your hands touching and teasing as You washed my hair ... commenting on the coconut shampoo and conditioner ... making jokes about piña-colada hair.

I could feel Your hands washing my body ... the soap on the

cloth making it feel so incredibly good ... soft ... slippery ... yet abrasive and relaxing ...

Your hands teasing and touching as You washed me. Washing every inch of my shaking body ...

You told me to lie back in the water and feel You as You explored my body. Hands found my breasts and pulled ... rubbed ... teased ... pinched ... and flicked a thumbnail over the sensitive tips of the nipples ... my pussy throbbed and ached ...

Fingers slid into the lips of my pussy ... teasing and tormenting the clit ... pinching it ... rolling it ... pulling on it ... making it throb ... swell ... ache for You ...

My body was so turned on ... as I imagined You stroking and touching me ... I heard You tell me to turn over ... You used my small vibe and inserted it anally ... turned it on high and then told me to sit up on it so it vibrated hard into me ... Then You used the power shower head ... running it all over my body ... all over my breasts ... especially on the nipples ... then lower till it hit my clit ...

I was moaning so loud and the feelings were so intense!

I could hear You telling me to open wider, to hold my pussy lips as You ran the water jet over my clit ... The muscles of my pussy contracting hard ...

The vibe in my ass was turned on high and it didn't take long before the two together made me come ... it was fast and hard ... the orgasm rolling over me in wave after wave. My body shook so hard ... the intensity making me scream Your name ... I came twice before I felt relieved and worn out enough to rest.

I could hear Your voice telling me to relax ... to feel You ... You told me You were holding me tight ... it was incredible ...

I finished up my bath and lay there a bit ... just relaxing and thinking of You ...

My hands running along my body...slowly touching... caressing...feeling the sensations...

I could hear Your soft voice whispering in my ear...calling me little one...telling me how pleased You are with me...that I was a good girl and made You so very happy...

My hands (Your hands) soon found my clit and began massaging it...pulling on it...teasing it...as the muscles contracted...I found my other vibe...my favourite dark blue with the ridges...and inserted it...I could feel You entering me...Feel You as You drove hard and deep into me...Your fingers found my nipples and squeezed and pulled them...

Turning the vibe on high...You used the shower head again on a lower setting...I could hear You moaning and feel You driving into me...My legs up on the sides of the tub...You drove me wild...As I came...I screamed Your name...over and over...as the intensity of one orgasm lightened...another would start building...

Your girl came five more times for You...

I lost all thought...all memory...there was nothing...just the feelings enveloping me hard and deep...

Then...Your soft kisses...Your hands on my nipples...the release as I came back down...slowly...the water surrounding my body...warming me...

The cold water waking me about half an hour later...I shivered as I got out of the tub and wrapped up in a huge warm towel...I lay on the couch about twenty minutes under a quilt getting warm...thinking of You...wishing so badly to hear Your voice...

I noticed the time and got up to get dressed...

I miss You, my Darlin' Sir...

Show and Tell

Abi, age 30
Heterosexual
Celibate
Master's degree
Writer
Northwest Cheshire, UK

I've had plenty of sexual experiences and I've had very adventurous boyfriends, so I was allowed to try out whatever took my fancy. I'm now celibate by choice, but I secretly delight in the knowledge of the things I know I can do.

In my fantasy I'm walking through an open garden and I meet my man. He's someone I know, but he's not very familiar. He's a big man physically. I smile and he slips his hands under my flowing blouse and grabs my nipples and starts rubbing and tugging at them. We don't kiss. I slip my hand into his trousers and grab his ass and pinch. There is a little bush with soft grass; it's big enough to hide us but people could still see if they looked. We stand behind it and I move my hand forwards and feel his cock; it's hard, thick and long. He bends his head and starts to suckle my breasts. I'm wearing a skirt and I push him down on the grass and unbuckle his pants just enough to release his cock. I'm very wet and I push my panties aside and mount his cock until it's deep inside and I start to ride him. His hands are clutching my ass but he's still suckling. He gets almost to the point where he climaxes, then I grab his balls and gently pull. He pushes me back on the grass with his cock still inside me, puts my hands together and holds them above my head with one hand while he continues to fondle my breasts with the other and sucks at them, pounding into me, fast then slow, then agonisingly slow and fast again. Just when we're about to climax, I get my hands free and grab his ass and hold him down into me till he empties his passion. We lie there for a while, then we stand up and kiss and he does up his trousers and I pull down my skirt, and we go our separate ways.

C E, age 36
Heterosexual
Single, occasionally sexually active
No children
Postgraduate degree
Writer/Photographer
New England, USA

A recurring theme in my fantasies is that of having my breasts – or the breasts of the fantasy character that can look quite different from me – manipulated in some way, sometimes roughly, usually while being penetrated. Another theme is being 'serviced' by multiple lovers at the same time. My current favourite fantasy emerged from a dream shared by an email pal. He dreamed that we met in Boston, in winter. I wore a long grey wool coat with nothing on underneath. Somehow we'd find ourselves in a secluded alley. And there, he'd push me against a wall and ravish me. The top button of the coat would come undone so that one breast would be exposed to the elements and to his fingers. As he fucked me, he would pinch that one nipple, until I came.

Marcie, age 34
Heterosexual
Live-in relationship/marriage
No children
College

Sales
Washington, USA

As I grow older, the more I want my fantasies to come true, to be forced out of my comfort zone – a little. My sex life would improve if my husband wasn't a prude. He is *very* plain in his tastes. He likes sex in one position, one way, and on Friday nights. It is pretty boring and old. It wasn't like this when we were dating, but it got this way after we were married. I tend to fantasise about having sex with someone I cannot see and don't know, someplace public with people who are watching. However, I don't know that they are watching until it's all over, and I'm left alone.

Lucy, age 21
Heterosexual
Steady relationship, not live-in
No children
Bachelor's degree
PR and Marketing Executive
Derbyshire, UK

I find the idea of being watched very erotic. I often fantasise about masturbating on a webcam with people paying to watch me use my vibrator. I also fantasise regularly about having a threesome with two men, and anal sex. My favourite current fantasy is having sex with a man when somebody is watching, but they don't know I know. Then they suddenly come and join in with us, and we all three have sex, with one man penetrating my vagina, and the other my anus.

Ginger, age 27
Heterosexual

Single, very sexually active
Degree
Journalist
London, UK

My boyfriend doing delicious things to my naked body normally does the trick for me. Occasionally I fantasise about public sex, and sometimes I fantasise about women, although not that often, as I'm a huge fan of the boys. I like confident, masculine men with big strong arms who make me feel like a rag doll. I've always had a strong sexual imagination, and I have an extremely high sex drive, but I'm also quite vanilla. I'm a hopeless romantic, so all my fantasies revolve around romance, sensuality, kisses and cuddles and, of course, one big fat gorgeous naked man! I read a lot of erotica for work, and I get turned on easily by most things, but ultimately thinking about my boyfriend if I haven't seen him for a while is enough to make me weak at the knees. Oh, except for Brad Pitt in *Thelma and Louise*. That gorgeous cowboy started off some amazing fantasies for me aged fourteen.

I have definitely become more confident as I've grown older, and hence have also developed more of a sexual imagination, but, as a hopeless romantic, my fantasies have always revolved around a loving and caring relationship. I watch more porn and read more erotica as part of my job, which I absolutely love, though ultimately my biggest turn-on is and has always been my imagination. I tend to use memory, so I usually think back to a really hot sexual experience I've already had with my boyfriend. Sometimes I just daydream about various sexual encounters we've had, or things I'd like to do with him. Usually it's quite straightforward, but occasionally I daydream that we're doing what we normally do, but there's lots of people watching. I like doggy-style, with him cupping my breasts and kissing my neck.

Name withheld, age 44
Heterosexual
Live-in relationship/marriage
Children
Teaching Assistant Certificate
Teaching Assistant
County Durham, UK

I didn't become aware of my sexuality until I was 38 years old when I met my second husband. I didn't enjoy sex at all and now I can't get enough. When I first met my second husband he was my son's maths teacher and married; I was divorced. We met for a drink one night and ended up having sex in the back of his car. It was the most mind-blowing experience I had ever had. I'd never had multi-orgasms before and they came one after another. He'd never had that effect on a woman before so it blew his mind too. I also gushed for the first time. Here is my fantasy.

I go into a bar to wait for someone that doesn't come. I order a drink. I see two men seated at a secluded booth. I catch them looking at me and I turn away. I look again and they are obviously talking about me. One man comes over to the bar and begins to make conversation. He asks me if I would like a drink and if I am waiting for anyone. I tell him that my friend has not turned up and he asks me if I'd like to join him and his friend at their booth. I decide to go for it and follow him over. They both introduce themselves and I do the same. The first man allows me to slide along the seat towards the other man so that I end up sitting between them. We make small talk for a while as the first man slowly slides his hand under the table and strokes my leg. I jump a little at the touch but really enjoy it. The other man sees my reaction and knows his friend has done something to me. Seeing that I have not reacted badly to it, he too places his hand under the table. They are both stroking my outer legs slowly up and down beneath the table where no one can see.

The feeling of two men touching me in a public place makes my heart beat faster and I want more. I begin to open my legs a little, which is easy as I'm wearing a short denim skirt. My legs push against each of the men's legs and they know what I'm doing. Instantly they move their hands and fingers towards my inner thighs and begin to stroke my soft skin. I can feel myself getting wet and rub myself very slowly and gently on the edge of the seat. The first man's fingers move towards my pussy which is throbbing, wanting attention from these two men. He slowly probes my pussy through my thong and eventually works his fingers into the side and, as an electric shock hits me, the other man steadies me with his other hand. They both smile at me and I allow myself to move slightly forwards, pushing against the first man's fingers, pressing them against my clit. The sensation is incredible and I want more, rocking back and forth. I can feel myself building towards a climax and so does the man. He pushes his fingers deep inside me, making me reach my orgasm, my throbbing wet pussy soaking his fingers. The other man steadies me again, holding me so no one will know what's happening, and he kisses me gently on the cheek. 'My turn,' he says, as they move their hands into opposite positions. I build again very slowly, but this time I take out both of the men's cocks and wank them slowly under the table as I reach another orgasm and another, the two men's hands working in unison, bringing me to climax after climax. I keep working on their throbbing cocks until I bring both of them to climax, their hot salty seed shooting all over my hands and the floor.

Helen, age 45
Heterosexual
Steady relationship, not live-in
College
Self-employed
London, UK

I used to be led and told what to do but now I'm very happy to instigate sex and to lead my partner into areas he hadn't thought of. My current partner is everything I've ever wanted (shame I didn't know this before) and if he talks dirty I'm in heaven. I am now old enough and confident enough to be able to enjoy whatever I want to do without worrying about the consequences. In my favourite fantasy my partner and I are parked in a busy car park at night, but the urge to make love overtakes us and we slowly undress each other, not worrying if anyone see or hears us. We're just wrapped up in the act of pleasuring each other.

Sonya, age 42
Bisexual
Live-in relationship/marriage
Children
Some college
Actress/Singer/Writer
Ontario, Canada

I'm turned on by being emotionally connected to my man, being able to be completely myself. I admit I like sex rough or anally, to be somewhat submissive or dominant, whatever my mood brings – and having him welcome all of me without judgement. Being a mother and knowing my body helped produce this other person makes me feel powerful and sexy too. I care much less now about how my body looks, what my face might look like when I'm aroused or coming, or what my man might think of me and my turn-ons. I don't obsess much anymore and therefore don't rob myself of a good time!

My fantasies tend to involve the following themes: the psychological process of a woman becoming aroused; the stages of sexuality and how they affect a woman throughout her maiden years to mother years; and the link and/or 'play' between the feeling of safety or danger in a sexual situation. My fantasies involving strangers hold me back because they are not safe. I am in a committed relationship now, and it takes several sexual encounters with someone to 'get me off' usually. I have always envied those women who could have the perfect satisfactory zipless fuck.

In my favourite fantasy I'm in a train, which is rocking and making me sleepy. I had forgotten how hard these commuter train benches are, old and wooden – German technology, with little comfort. The sun is setting and my eyes are tired of racing to catch the scenery, one tree and church steeple at a time, so I close them for a while. I am somewhere between Paris and Munich.

I kick my sandals off and raise my legs. I tuck my heels close to my bum, with my knees pointing upwards and my toes hanging off the edge of the bench. It feels good to stretch the front of my thighs this way. I'm wearing a short skirt and a thong and I'm alone in the car, so I feel it's safe to do this. I rest my head back and dream of the man I've just left behind.

It's a horrible thing to admit that I miss his cock more than the rest of him, but it's true. And he's left me wet, with a little of him and a lot of my own juices. As my legs relax a little and my cunt opens slightly, I get a waft of our pleasure. It makes me remember how he slid first two, then three, then four fingers in me, so slow and gentle. It's shocking to know I not only could accommodate so much of his hand, but I also relished the sensation of being so stretched open and filled. When his cock followed after his fist, I slowly clenched and closed around it, grateful for the relative softness and curve it offered by then, grateful for having such control over my cunt and proud of its parlour tricks. What a marvellous instrument it is.

He had rocked inside of me like this train, languidly but with a quiet and steady vigour. He stayed still and eager when my eyes flew open and demanded he look at me as I came. It made me come harder to know he was seeing contradiction on my face, with my pleasure and vulnerability revealed all at once. It was the only time I had ever really let him in.

I feel my thong getting wetter and realise it won't be long before I'm dripping. I open my eyes. On the bench in front of me is a man. I hadn't heard him come in and now he's gazing at me with a smile and half-closed eyes. He's not handsome but strangely compelling, as he is rough and sexual. He's bull-necked with a fighter's face and a confidence that comes from within. He's well-dressed in a nice suit, his muscles bulging through the fine fabric.

I stay perfectly still, unsure of what to do next. He doesn't move or change his expression. I don't feel threatened by him. I am simply embarrassed, as any attempt to pull myself together at this point would be comical. Then I find a strange freedom in this moment. I decide to play with him.

I open my legs a bit more and inch forwards slightly, causing my thong to be pulled and bury itself in my cleft, and I feel my outer lips push forwards and engulf it. They slowly fold over the small strip of fabric, and this gives me a thrill. I feel a new surge of wetness.

I see his eyes drop down and look at my exposed lips as he shifts in his seat. He adjusts his cock with his hand and looks back up at me, and his smile disappears. I can almost hear the blood rushing to his dick. I drop my gaze to his crotch and his hands. They are huge. His fingers are long and thick and he has flat wide fingertips. I look back at him and jut my chin forwards, a silent dare for him to pull his cock out or at least a dare of some kind. He smiles again.

I hoist myself up a little and, keeping my feet up and my legs bent, I hook my thong with my thumb and pull it aside. With the pressure of having sat this way for some time, both sets of lips and my clit are engorged. Everything is protruding a little. And my hole is open a bit, I can feel cool air there. I drop my head back again, close my eyes and, wrapping my arms under my legs just behind my ankles, I pull my cunt lips apart as wide as I can. I tilt my head up again and look to see his reaction. His mouth is hanging open and his hand is shaking as it unzips his pants. He suddenly seems to remember to use his other hand to help himself, as if one side of his brain is not working in tandem with the other. I have a small moment of satisfaction when I think of how visual men are and how powerful a cunt can be when used this way. I now know what all the fuss is about with owning your sexuality. I smile.

He takes out a thick meaty cock and, with the first thrust into his fist, the foreskin rolls back to reveal a huge bulbous head. It sticks out at the top of his fist a good four inches. This penis looks like it belongs on some sort of animal. Its mushroom head is a vicious shade of purple. It's so obscene it turns me on. He seems content to stay there and watch me from this short distance, with his eyes on my cunt and his hand pumping his cock. He is sweating now and breathing heavily. I put my feet on the floor and scoot forwards a little. I reach between my legs and start rubbing my clit. I dip my fingers in, first one, then two, and wet my clit this way repeatedly. I stop rubbing now and then and spread myself, enjoying the feeling of being examined by this stranger. I feel like an object, a porno, as he is not even looking at my face. It makes me feel safer somehow.

My clit is so swollen and my juices are running off the bottom of me. His cock is slick now too, and makes a sticky wet sound with every stroke. His breathing is punctuated by a small grunting noise. He leans forwards and for a moment my pleasure is suspended. I am terrified of what he may do next. He leans in close, his face inches away from my cunt, and starts sniffing. He smells me for a beat and then leans back again, licks his lips and pumps furiously on his dick. I start stroking again and begin to feel the tingle, that watery feeling in my legs and belly and I know I'm going to come soon. Just as I throw my head back and start to come, I hear his come – *splat, splat* – on the floor between us. The sound is so vulgar. I feel it splatter my feet, my ankles. I ride my wave for as long as I can and finally shudder to a stop. I start to laugh. This uncontrollable giggle bubbles up from within me and I start to laugh hard. I want to share this moment with my man here but when I lift my head up and open my eyes, I find him gone.

Three's Not a Crowd

Name withheld, age 21
Heterosexual
Steady relationship, not live-in
No children
College
Graphic Designer
New England, USA

I have a current fantasy of travelling with my boyfriend to a Latin American location by train – which is not really possible, but, oh well – with a hot tour guide (girl or boy). Along the journey, the tour guide discovers my boyfriend and me making love in our sleeping car. (S)he does not turn away and instead joins us in the small bed. Said tour guide 'tours' our conjoined bodies, tasting and caressing each body part with intense curiosity. During the trip we continue to play with our new friend, discovering more and more about our adventurous side through trips into the Amazon, the hot sands of Brazil and hiking through mountains.

Rach, age 32
Heterosexual
Single, moderately sexually active
Children
Education and Occupation unknown
Brisbane, Australia

The best sex I ever had was after a long weekend of drinking and camping on the beach. I came home and jumped under the cool shower with my ex, and had him fuck me up the arse while standing up. I'm turned on by having a guy whisper in my ear all the things he'd like to do to me and how, seeing him pull himself over me, then bending me over and fucking me. I fantasise several times a day. In my favourite fantasy I am being held down by two good-looking men and they're both having their way with me.

Jacquie, age 44
Bisexual
Single, very sexually active
Children
College
Receptionist
Tasmania, Australia

My favourite fantasy is three men playing with me; on all levels, no holds barred, nothing stopped, want it, do it. The only thing holding me back from fulfilling it is finding the men who will play together. They have so many hang-ups!

Naz, age 29
Bisexual
Single, very sexually active
No children
Postgraduate degree
Journalist
West Midlands, UK

I fantasise regularly about shagging several of my friends and we all flirt outrageously although nothing has happened. I think we're all up for it, but they're a married couple and, while my fantasies, daydreams and even a couple of memorable nights where I've woken up gasping and wet from dreams that make my toes curl, tell me it would be amazing, in the back of my mind I'm concerned enough to hold back because I don't want to do anything that would damage their marriage or, indeed, our friendships. It can't stop a girl from dreaming, though.

In my fantasy she's gorgeous. She's got the kind of plump luscious lips that set my mind racing with very rude thoughts, stunning cornflower blue eyes and a mane of red hair that falls to her shoulders. As I look at her, she tucks a wayward strand behind her ear, her hand trembling slightly and, although she's smiling, her eyes betray a little wariness. I guess standing naked in front of someone you've never met before does that.

In my peripheral vision I see my fuck buddy Andy take a step back and sit down on the arm of the sofa. She turns her head skittishly at the movement, her hair falling back in front of her face. She moves her hand, but I am faster, and, as I gently tuck the silken strand back behind her ear, she shyly smiles her thanks. I feel my nipples harden in response. God, she's gorgeous.

I stroke her hair, calming her, and move closer. I hear Andy shift slightly to get a better view of what's about to happen, but this time I don't turn around, and neither does she. We're looking intently at each other, waiting to see what happens next. I half expect him to intervene, this is his scene after all, but it seems this is our dance and ours alone. For now.

I stroke her hair for a long time. The only sound in the room is our breathing, the only movement my hand stroking her head, relaxing her. Slowly, as if not to break the spell, I lean forwards to kiss her.

She tastes of strawberry lip balm and mint. To start with, her only reaction is a whispered sigh, swallowed between our joined mouths. But as I start to pull away to break the kiss, she moves closer, anchoring her fingers into my hair and pulling my head back. Suddenly our tongues are vying for possession. She holds me in position and sucks hard on my bottom lip, and I smile as I think what she will be like with her mouth on my cunt. She might be another submissive girl and she's obviously nervous, but there's attitude there. I like her.

She moves her hands up my body, tentatively touching the underside of my breast, her soft cool fingers tracing a lazy path along my skin as our tongues tangle. I move my hand to her breast to stroke the delicate edge of her puckered coral nipple. But, before I can fully touch it, we're being dragged apart.

We both blink, confused, unable to focus for a second. Her pupils are dilated with her arousal and I wonder fleetingly if mine look the same. Our ragged breathing slows and Andy's smiling face comes back into focus.

He's standing between us like a referee between two prize fighters in the ring, holding a wrist in each hand like a vice. 'I'm pleased you're getting on so well,' he says. 'But I don't want you getting distracted before we play a little game.'

My face obviously betrays my frustration at the abrupt end of our touching as he releases her wrist – he's obviously not risking releasing mine yet – to pinch my nipple, hard enough to be as much in warning as in play.

'Don't worry, you'll get a chance to continue. In fact, I think you're really going to enjoy this game. Not only is it fun to play but I'll fuck the winner while the other watches.' He idly runs a finger around my nipple before pinching it again. 'Of course, whoever loses is going to be left frustrated for a long time since they'll be attending our every need for the duration.'

Suddenly my competitive juices are flowing almost as freely as my cunt juices. I want one mouth at each breast, teeth nipping at my nipples, I want her between my legs, hot mouth on my clit while Andy fucks me until I'm about to pass out from the number of orgasms wrung from my shuddering body. As the images flash through my mind like a porn movie, I become resolute.

Whatever this game is, I'm going to ensure that I win it. No matter what.

But Andy's smiling knowingly. He moves to the table to pick up something I can't see, and it makes me uneasy. It's like he's read my mind and is amused to know this isn't going to be as easy as I hope.

He gestures for us to lie on the floor, and manoeuvres us around so we're lying in a sixty-niner. I begin to smile as I see how close I am to the glistening strawberry red curls of her cunt – this game isn't going to be a hardship at all. Then I see the ribbon. Andy ties my hands together and then, with a longer piece of ribbon, binds them to her thighs, effectively leaving my head clamped between her legs and her unable to squirm away. As he moves down and ties her the same way between my thighs I cautiously test the bonds – it may be ribbon but there's no give in it and the knots are tight. Until he chooses to cut us free there's really nowhere to go.

He sits down on the sofa in front of us, master of all he surveys, and we both turn to look at him, our heads framed with the other's thighs.

'It's really very simple and, by the look of how much fun you were both having earlier, it's not going to be a hardship. I want you to lick each other out. Gently, hard, mashing your faces deep into each other's cunts or nibbling the clit.'

She gasps slightly at the bluntness of Andy's order, her breath on my mound making me shudder. 'You can do it however you like. But the objective is to make the other girl come. Again. And again. And again. The winner is the one who makes the other orgasm most.' Andy's smiling down at me and I know why he's so amused.

'Which may be a problem if you're especially sensitive after an orgasm and unable to squirm away from someone intent on making you come again.'

Fuck. I'm already so wet I can feel my juices running down my inner thighs. Being tied down, licking out a stunning girl, Andy watching the whole thing, is making me so stupidly horny that I already know the odds aren't in my favour. And that's before he shows us the riding crop.

'And if I don't think you're putting in enough effort with each other, or if you begin to tire, I'll swat you with this until you speed up again. Now begin.'

He sits back to enjoy the show.

And as I feel her tongue lick along my already slick pussy

lips I know I'm lost. I think I'm about to find out you can have too much of a good thing.

And it's going to be a bloody amazing ride.

Rena, age 30
Heterosexual
Single, occasionally sexually active
No children
High School diploma
Retail
Ohio, USA

I think the first time I became aware of myself sexually I was eleven or twelve. My uncle used to get adult books and magazines and I was a child who would read anything, so I would sneak in and read them. The ones that I read the most almost always involved oral sex. Whether it was a man/woman or woman/woman it didn't matter. Those stories always seemed to be the ones that turned me on the most. It was by reading those stories that I discovered what I could do for myself to make me feel good. Right now the things that really get the juices going are girl/girl scenes. I'm not a lesbian, but the women in these scenes really get into what they are doing, getting each other off. In the last few books I've read, the sexual scenes that I liked were the alpha males who took control in the bedroom. A few of the scenes drifted towards submissive/dominant, but not to the extreme.

As for the best sex I've ever had – it's been so long since I've had sex I'm not sure that I can remember! Let's see . . . I was seventeen. I was sneaking out to be with my neighbour. Since we were both sneaking, we almost always ended up at the graveyard. I was feeling particularly horny that night and could not wait to meet with him. As a teenage boy, he knew nothing about foreplay so most of the times we were together were over pretty quick. This night was different. He was never much of a kisser so we usually skipped all that. Once we got to our 'spot', he slowly unsnapped my shirt and took his time exploring my tits. He rolled the nipples between his fingers, even bent down to lick and suck on them. He'd never done that before. While he continued to lick and suck on my tits, one of his hands travelled down between my legs. He rubbed me back and forth through my pants a little before unzipping them so that he could touch me skin to skin. He always knew where to find my clit, but he never touched or rubbed me long enough to satisfy me. While his hands were busy in my pants, mine were working on removing his shirt. This action got in the way of his mouth on my breasts, but that was fine. What I really wanted to do was go down on him.

The first time I had ever done that to him I had been really shy and now that I had a little experience under his belt, it became something that I enjoyed doing to him. Once his shirt was off, I moved to his pants and by now he figured out what I was trying to do and helped me. He took his hand out of my pants and yanked his own down to his ankles. Down on my knees, I pulled him free of his boxers and proceeded to lick his shaft from top to bottom. I held and caressed his balls with my hand while I used my tongue all over his dick. When his hand squeezed my shoulder, I knew that's when he wanted me to suck him fully into my mouth. He wasn't very big, so taking him all the way to my throat was not a problem. As I bobbed my head up and down on him, I'd swirl my tongue around the head and suck really hard on my way back up (one time his dick made a popping noise when he pulled out of my mouth after I sucked real hard, we had been trying to do that again ever since . . . to no avail). I quit moving my head so that he could thrust into my mouth at his own speed and, when his hips started to move a little too fast, I knew he was close to coming. Pulling back a little, I started to lick him again, letting his orgasm hold off a bit.

Now I was ready to fuck him. We would do it from behind more often than not, and this night was no exception. No matter how many times we had sex, I always liked the feel of him sliding into me. He reached around to grab my tits and started thrusting real slow. Once he set his pace, I started to thrust back into him, trying to get him deeper inside me. I put my hand between my legs so that I could feel his dick sliding in and out of me and play with my clit a little. Then he did something that he had never done before. He moved my hand out of the way and used his own hand to play with my clit. It felt so good my knees started to get a little weak. While he played with my clit, he quit thrusting and buried himself to the hilt inside me and just started to roll his hips without pulling out too much. This combined with his fingers on my clit just pushed me over the edge. I had never had an orgasm like that before. When my muscles clenched around his dick, he let his orgasm go and both of us started thrusting like crazy until we couldn't stand anymore. I've had some pretty good experiences since then, but that stands out as one of the best.

I usually fantasise about threesomes with myself and two men, someone unattainable that I would never meet in the daily course of my life. I've always wondered what it would be like to be penetrated at the same time by both of them. I've seen it done in adult movies and ever since I've wondered what the feeling of that kind of fulfilment would be like. To be with two men whose sole goal was my pleasure first, to have my body worshipped and loved ...

Debbie, age 44
Bisexual
Celibate
Postgraduate student
Clinic Manager/Poet
London, UK

I fantasise about lying on my back on the bed, my head hanging off the edge and being fucked in the mouth (a backwards blow job); sixty-niners; sitting on his face – often with another woman involved, i.e., her kissing me at same time or me licking her cunt at the same time, or him fucking me and licking her, or him fucking her with me and her kissing!

Rhonda, age 29
Bisexual
Single, moderately sexually active
Steady relationships, not live-in
No children
Doctorate degree
Professor
Ohio, USA

I have two fantasies. I'll start with the most recent, most embarrassing to admit, hence the reason I have to write it out. I was told the fetish is called 'furries'. Apparently these are individuals who enjoy dressing up and/or engaging in sexual activity with another dressed in a furry costume, i.e., fuzzy rabbit, chicken, dog, etc., costumes. My most recent fantasy involves an unknown beautiful woman in a bunny costume, her breasts exposed through the costume (via cut-out holes), and a boyfriend and me engaging in a threesome with the bunny-costumed woman. We engage in intercourse and, while both massaging the unknown woman's breasts, we climax. Repeat this scenario, but with her rear exposed also, and actually engaging in intercourse with the woman. All of this is, of course, being videotaped.

True tale: my editor, no name here, and I have had this banter-nip-and-dodge routine for some time now. I find him cute and his wife adorable. My editor and I did not always like each other; in fact, we could not, initially, stand each other. In my fantasy, time soldiers on, we realise we respect each other as writers, as talent on and off screen and, oh, right, of course, we kinda dig each other. And he digs his wife. And I dig his wife. They dig me. While this could easily be a night of debauchery, I want to try and maintain *some* professional decorum, so I allow myself a little fun – his wife paddles me, he bends us both over and paddles us, and I make out with his wife little. However, this all happened *after* we met to discuss some notes – while alone, briefly, out of the fucking blue – or he's just that good at reading people, because I am a damn great actress – he grabs me, flips me over his knee, quickly pulls up my dress, pulls down my panties, spanks my bare bottom a few times, pulls the panties up, the dress down, and flips me back over. Estimated time-frame: twenty seconds. I am amazed, flushed, excited, and proceed to giggle and touch myself over it for weeks to come.

Rosemary, age 49
Heterosexual
Single, moderately sexually active
Children
Master's degree
Writer/Tutor
Bristol, UK

Being tied up by my brothers was the first time when I felt sexually excited! I lost my virginity in the open air with snow on the ground. I find sex outdoors extremely exciting. I love the feel of fresh air blowing about my nether regions. Erotic writing in books probably does it more than film, which is horribly choreographed. Porn films do excite me, but in a guilty kind of way as I don't really like the way women are usually exploited in them.

What turns me on are masculine men with big cocks who are cock-sure of themselves and who have a witty, knowing, boyish charm about them; and being surprised and fucked by men I didn't even know fancied me, especially when it feels like uncontrollable lust – out of doors, in cars, in alleyways before anyone sees, being taken over by the moment. Dressing up as a naughty schoolgirl or tart, or turning up for a date in a very public place wearing nothing underneath or just underwear, stockings and suspenders, is another turn-on. I'd love to have a threesome, but haven't found any men I fancy who'd want to do that. The children hold me back, as I don't have sex in the house if they're there, especially as I like to be noisy.

My favourite fantasy starts off slowly with a big strong man who's probably slightly unshaven. He begins by whispering that he wants my big juicy cunt and that I'm *sooo* sexy, etc. He takes off my clothes – no, not all of them – I have my underwear on. He doesn't have time to take off all his clothes – just his trousers – but when he unleashes his cock it's huge and throbbing and dribbling a little come on the end. He shows me his huge cock and I'm wriggling excitedly, but he doesn't let me have it yet. He doesn't put on a condom. He teases me by rubbing around and around the outside of my vagina while I'm pleading with him to fuck me, fuck me hard. He pulls my panties to one side and enters me – deeply – I gasp, he holds off, looking down into my eyes, then begins to fuck me slowly,

slowly. I've got my hands on his big muscular arse, and there's someone watching. Oh, there's someone watching. I want to escape, but he's got me pinned down by the arms; he takes out some rope, or it might be ribbon, to tie my arms to the bedstead. But there's someone watching. Someone's watching – it's another man and he's pulling on his dick and watching as the big man rides me hard and deep and good and I come and come and come. He comes inside me and I can feel his lovely big cock spurting inside me. 'You're a very dirty girl,' he whispers, and the other guy comes over and fucks me too, and I come again. Then the first guy returns and fucks me, but pulls out before he comes and then shoots all over my tits. My hands are loose and I rub the come into my tits as they're both now all over me.

Beth, age 45
Heterosexual
Single, occasionally sexually active
Children
B S degree
Recruiter
California, USA

I really like multiple males. I don't see why I can't have two men in my bed . . . well, other than the fact that I don't even seem to have one at the moment, but hey . . .

My current favourite fantasy is that this brilliant chemist I know invites me over, planning to seduce me, and a friend of his just happens by while we're having some rather normal sex. It gets progressively less realistic from there – probably to do with too much abstinence. His friend has dark hair and blue eyes, the chemist has blond hair and brown eyes – a fun mix. I end up moving in with both of them and having a couple of kids, one with each (I don't know why, but it's part of the fantasy), some pets, and envious neighbours who either wish I was their girlfriend or else hate me because they want another man in their relationship. Weird, huh? Or not, I guess, as it seems to be a recurring theme in other books and such.

Ruth, age 35
Heterosexual
Live-in relationship/marriage
No children
Degree
Health and Safety Manager
East Midlands, UK

My fantasy is written as a short story. My lover Carl and I are in Paris. It's a cold day, and when he comes to pick me up from my apartment he devours me hungrily with his eyes, taking in my knee-high black leather boots, tightly fitted black polo-neck top, straight black skirt that ends a couple of inches above my knee, my black stockings, my long camel-coloured woollen coat, and my long blonde hair curling around my face and over my shoulders. I know he is envisaging the tops of my stockings edged in lace, the fine black satin-and-lace panties and bra that I have on, and the matching suspender belt. He leans in towards me as if to kiss me but stops before he touches my lips. Bending slightly, he slowly runs his hand up the inside of my skirt, up my leg from the top of my boot, savouring the sensation of the change from leather to nylon to skin, finally bringing his hand up to the satin of my panties, letting his thumb rest over my sensitive bud and his fingers over my pussy. I moan lightly and he smiles, knowing he could take me right now if he so chooses. He kisses me lightly and takes his hand away.

Today we are going lingerie shopping to a small but elite boutique in the Latin Quarter, where I have a private account. They sell the most exquisitely beautiful lingerie in all of Paris and they provide a service whereby they close the shop for private viewings for account customers. On our arrival at the shop, the owner, Brigitte, closes the door behind us, locking it and putting up a sign discouraging other shoppers. I know her well, but this is Carl's first visit with me and I see that he is taken aback by her elegance and stunning beauty, and I remember the breathtaking effect she had on me when I first met her. She is tall, slim, graceful, and immaculately dressed in an ivory silk long-sleeved blouse, a straight black pencil skirt to the knee, flesh-coloured stockings, and high-heeled black shoes. Her hair is a rich chestnut colour and is tied back in a smooth pleat. Her eyes are green and dance with delight as she welcomes us to her domain, kissing us warmly on each cheek.

Brigitte takes our coats from us and I see her favourably appraise my lover, taking in his long legs, tall 6' 2" frame, broad chest and shoulders, dark colouring and lovely brown eyes. I smile, content to be there with such a sexy man.

We are told that the shop is ours for the rest of the afternoon. We spend a leisurely hour looking around, choosing our favourite items among the delicate, the sensual, and the most overtly sexual of undergarments. We choose twelve sets in total and other items that we find sexy including French knickers, stockings, suspenders, tights, corsets and basques.

We are then taken over to the changing room, which is large and mirrored and has a thick cream carpet and sumptuous drapery hanging in ivory, gold and deep red. We're shown to a large leather sofa and given rich coffee to drink. I can see Carl looking around in wonder at our fine surroundings, unaware of the lovely show that is about to unfold. I have not told him that part of the service is that everything we choose is modelled for us so that we can both sit back and decide. I have seen this many times and it's always a pleasantly arousing experience, so I look forward to the effect it's going to have on him. However, I instantly realise that we are getting a little extra service today as Brigitte brings all the garments in and slowly begins to undress. The change of clothing is not normally carried out in front of the customer. My beautiful man looks at me and smiles in a way that lets me know he is agreeably surprised. I can only nod as I'm also slightly taken aback, realising that we are in for a real treat.

Something in the mood is different today; usually Brigitte and I make idle conversation while she undresses behind a curtain, but today, as she unhurriedly removes her blouse and skirt, she locks eye contact with both of us, smiling slightly, none of us saying a word. She stands before us in her beautiful ivory silk patterned bra and brief waterfall French knickers and gracefully bends to remove her shoes and stockings. Then she slowly removes her bra to reveal small but perfectly shaped pert breasts with mid-brown erect nipples. On removing her panties, she stands to her full height in front of us and pauses, letting us clearly see that she is cleanly shaven, before retrieving the first of the items she's to try on for us. I have my hand resting on Carl's muscular thigh and as I feel the material of his trousers move, I realise that the vision of this stunning woman is as arousing for him as it is for me. He can't take his eyes off her, and he finds the fact that she hasn't stopped gazing at me so erotic. He looks at me then and notices that I too am looking directly at her; he sees that my lips are slightly parted and I'm gently biting the corner of my lower lip, my breathing a little more rapid than normal.

He turns his attention back to Brigitte as she reaches for the first of the garments – a gorgeous satin-and-lace set in coffee and ivory. Once she's fully dressed, complete with matching suspender belt, stockings and shoes, she then walks towards us and stands a little way in front so that we can admire the effect of the rich material against her faultless skin. Then, turning away, she returns to the centre of the room and lets us admire her from a distance.

With every change of luxurious lingerie, she slowly and tantalisingly removes each item and pauses for us to take in her perfect frame before adorning herself with another item. As she approaches to show us the lingerie, each time she's standing closer and closer. She is now not only looking at me, but spending long moments gazing at Carl too. The grace of her movements and her unfaltering stare is truly hypnotic and we are both spellbound. I can feel my nipples harden and my pussy is aching with desire at the sight of such elegant beauty. Her eyes drop briefly to his crotch and I see them twinkle as she notes his trousers are straining where his hardened cock is desperate to be set free.

When she has worked her way through all the items, she puts our final choice on: a very sheer white bra and panties edged with white satin. The effect against her olive skin is incredible. She makes her way towards us, feline in her move-ments, until she's standing so close that her knee is touching mine. She reaches down and takes my hand and gently pulls me towards her, encouraging me to feel the garments she's wearing and look more closely at them. I run my fingers over the sheer fabric, over the top line of the panties and dropping my fingers until they are an inch above where her beautiful sex slit begins. Moving up her body, I run my finger along the bottom of the bra, stopping in the middle of her breast and then running my thumb upwards over her fully erect nipple. With my other hand I caress her neckline, reaching around to the back of her hair, releasing it from its tidy pleat and letting her lush thick mane fall down around her shoulders. She puts her hand into my hair and pulls my face towards her, stopping briefly to look at my sexy lover; she then turns back towards me and kisses me deeply. Carl looks at us frozen in place, struck by the contrast of me clad entirely in black against her in the finest, flimsiest, pure white lingerie. The contrast is staggering and his proud cock twitches uncontrollably.

Slowly this divine creature pulls away from me, leading me by the hand and beckoning for him to follow us. She takes us over to one side of the dressing room, where behind one of the heavy curtains is a hidden door. She opens it and we follow her through. We find ourselves in an opulent bedroom, with a large bed at its centre made up with ivory satin sheets. The room also boasts several comfortable chairs and sheer chiffon hanging all around the walls, softening the edges and making it feel like a dreamscape.

She leads me over to the middle of the room next to the bed and slowly begins removing my clothes, kissing each part of my flesh that's being exposed as she works her way down my body. Finally we are standing together only in our lingerie, hers so pure and white and mine so black, and we kiss intensely, our tongues fucking and gently biting each other's lips, our breath shallow and our skin deliciously warm on each other. We lie on the bed together and continue kissing, hands running over each other's bodies. She pulls away from me slowly and we both turn to look at my man – he needs no more invitation and immediately begins to remove his clothes until he's naked. We see his beautifully engorged cock, and Brigitte moans delightedly when he joins us on the bed. The three of us spend a long time kissing and touching, with Carl slowly removing our undergarments, tasting and licking us as he does so.

Gently, Brigitte and I lay Carl back on the pillows, and between us we begin to cover his body with our mouths, working our way towards his lovely thick long cock. My mouth is already desperate to taste him and eager to lick away the pre-come that I can see oozing from the end of his delicious shaft. Together she and I lick his length slowly, delectably making our way up to the swollen purple head. Our lovely friend then moves back down Carl's shaft to concentrate on licking and suckling on his balls, while I take the shiny head of his dick into my mouth and watch as his eyes involuntarily roll backwards in absolute delight. She and I continue to please him, changing positions, but continually ensuring he's licked and sucked into a frenzy. We perform on him very slowly and deliberately, making his orgasm as prolonged as possible, until eventually Brigitte slides him into her mouth. Fucking her beautiful face, he can hold back no longer and shoots his hot cream deep into her throat. She pulls away and comes to me, kissing me deeply, sharing with me Carl's warm salty juices, letting me taste his sexiness and making me long for so much more.

Leaving him to luxuriate in his orgasmic glow, she and I fall to the bed together beside him, still kissing before I pull away and turn myself slowly around, kissing the length of her beautiful body until I reach her musky, moist sex. I can't wait to have her and I immediately bury my face in her cunt, making her moan deeply. She follows my lead and slides her rigid tongue into my soaking inner hole, but I tell her to take it easy and not to let me come. My handsome man raises himself on his elbow beside us and watches as we tongue-fuck each other's pussies right in front of him and he delicately strokes our skin, mesmerised by the act of sensual passionate love between us. Working on her lips and tight hole with my fingers and licking and sucking her clit, I take my time and gradually I bring her to an intense climax.

As we finish I can feel Carl's cock alert again, prodding and twitching against my back. I feel a desperate need to have him filling my wet sex slit and, slowly pulling him to the edge of the bed, I have him sit there while I turn my back on him and lower myself backwards onto his once-again hard length. He opens his legs, making mine spread even wider; as he does so Brigitte kneels between my man's knees and begins to lick my clit as I slide slowly up and down his rock-hard shaft. He reaches around and tenderly fondles my breasts while she works at my clitoris, and his cock twitches uncontrollably as I move on top of him. My orgasm isn't long in coming and, as I climax, my juices flow freely downwards from me, soaking his balls. Brigitte bends further and licks and sucks my lover's balls, taking in all my come while I fuck him harder, gathering speed and thrusting more deeply. It's not long before his hot salty love juice explodes deep inside me.

Our hostess raises herself from her knees and helps me to stand with her, again kissing me and running her hands over my ample tits and curves. I leave her standing, but pull Carl from the bed to kneel in front of her while I circle around behind her and also drop to my knees. Once there he doesn't waste any time in starting to work on her shaven wet sex; her lips are swollen and her bud enlarged. I separate her lovely arse cheeks and with my tongue begin to trace a line down the crack of her bum over her butthole and down towards her sex, where I find Carl's tongue busily at work. I work my way back up to her lovely tight asshole and begin running my tongue around the edge and then I push my tongue inside her deepest, most intimate, depths. She moans and bucks on top of us, her hot juices running from her as my lover concentrates on her clit, holding her lips apart with his fingers, and I slide two fingers inside her dripping pussy, tongue-fucking her arse. Her climax is long and noisy as she grinds on top of us, her hair dangling in tendrils around her lovely sweaty face, being more fully fucked than ever before. Her legs tremble and give way, and the three of us fall to the floor, panting and replete in post-sexual pleasure.

As we leave Brigitte we tell her that we'll take all of the items she's shown to us, and she assures me they will be delivered to my apartment the next day.

Carl and I walk back out into the cold day. Still hot from the arousal of our afternoon, we are on a high. But I still feel as if it ended without one final burst for either of us so, dragging him down the side of a building, I tell him I'm going to fuck him again. Instantly his cock leaps to attention and, out of sight of the road, he lifts me, pinning me against the wall, yanking my skirt up to my thighs. Ripping my panties from me, he releases his beautiful length and buries his cock in me harder and deeper than before, pumping away at my cunt like he never has before. Our climaxes come fast and furious, borne of extreme arousal, need and desperation.

We leave the alley hand in hand, laughing and sated, happy to be in Paris with all her hidden pleasures.

Jacqueline, age 36
Bisexual
Live-in relationship/marriage
Children
High School diploma
Teaching Assistant
Suffolk, UK

The fantasy that I enjoy the most would be one that involves myself and my partner, and would incorporate elements of our real sex life, including swinging. I imagine us in the Jacuzzi of the spa that we go to occasionally. It is full of couples and one beautiful blonde in her mid-30s. My partner and I are relaxing, leaning back against the side of the Jacuzzi watching couples and small groups getting together, kissing and fucking each other both in the Jacuzzi and on the side. I am feeling very horny as he slips his arm around me and fondles my pierced nipple. I can feel someone's foot sliding up my leg and stroking the inside of my thigh. I look across and realise that the blonde I noticed earlier is the owner of the leg. I smile at her and she takes the initiative and comes over and slides in next to me. As I turn to kiss my partner, my tits rise up out of the bubbles and she leans down to take one of my nipples into her mouth and sucks hard. I can feel myself starting to come and my partner can feel my body tense so he slides his hand down to my pussy and rubs on my clit. Almost instantaneously I come and even in the water it's possible to feel that I am gushing.

My new lady friend takes hold of my hand and suggests that the three of us go upstairs to one of the rooms. As we climb the stairs, she moves towards a private room, but I have other ideas and lead us into a large room with soft lighting and a huge round bed. The three of us settle ourselves down on the bed and I turn to kiss the lady, sliding my hands up and down her curvy body. My partner lies behind me, kissing my shoulders and running his hands over me in reflection of how I touch her. The three of us are so engrossed that we don't hear the door open or notice the people who have walked in and are settling themselves on chairs around the bed. By now, I am aching to taste her and to feel him inside me. I turn her onto her back and raise her legs up so that I can push my face into her wet shaven pussy. I love the taste of her and enjoy licking her clit and sliding my pierced tongue in and out of her. She bucks her hips up and down against my face, and I enjoy the sweetness of her. It's not long before I feel my partner slide his huge hard cock inside me. The first thrust is so powerful that I'm pushed even further against her, which she obviously enjoys because she pulls my head into her with both hands. I love the taste of her but I want her to fulfil a long time fantasy of mine. I pull away from her and she slides around so that her face is upside-down against mine. We kiss for a while and then I whisper into her ear my unfulfilled fantasy. She says nothing, but slides further down underneath me until she reaches my clit. Now I am in ecstasy; not only do I have the man that I love, and who satisfies me like no one else ever has before, sliding in and out of my pussy with his hard thick cock, but I also have a beautiful buxom blonde licking and sucking on my clit. It feels amazing and just gets better when I reach down and suck on her nipples.

As I glance up before changing to suck the other nipple, I notice the people watching us. This excites me even more because I know that as much as they might want to join us it isn't going to happen; this is about the three of us, no one else. I just know that I am going to gush and squirt again and just as I'm about to explode, my partner pulls his cock out of my tight wet pussy and I gush into her mouth with the force of a waterfall. It obviously wasn't what she was expecting, but despite a few splutters she takes it all down and swallows. My partner is kneeling on the bed wanking on his cock and looking gorgeous with beads of sweat trickling down his chest. I pull her towards me and ask her to kneel before him with her hands behind her back and her mouth open; meanwhile I lie down underneath him and open my mouth so that I can take his balls into my mouth and suck on them and lick them, flicking the end of my tongue against the base of his cock. I just know that he's going to explode all over her face when he comes and I know that she is going to be shocked with the amount of come. It's obvious that he is in control because, despite the fact that he's clearly on the edge, he is holding it back and savouring the power. When I feel his balls go hard I know it's not going to be long before he comes, and sure enough I feel the thrusts and hear her shocked squeal as he comes all over her face. I slide out and kneel in front of her and hold the back of her head. She looks at me and I pull her towards me and kiss her deeply, feeling the warm sticky come rub off onto my face and into my mouth. It's amazing.

Gillian, age 44
Bisexual
Live-in relationship/marriage
Children
College degree
Writer/Mother
Somerset, UK

The first time I realised I might be bi was while staying at a friend's, where we shared a double bed. She had breasts, which I didn't as yet. She was thirteen, with a fully formed womanly body. Her areolas were large and dark, with large protruding nipples – something she disliked but I loved. When she was asleep I would touch her.

I like going to swinging parties. I don't often go with any men but normally just enjoy watching others or watching my husband with other women, either singly or in a group. I also like watching my husband masturbate, especially when he thinks I'm not watching him. If I'm out I will look at girls and sometimes see someone who's really nice-looking and has lovely shaped tits. The girl who does my eyebrows is like that. She told me out of the blue that she likes doing full body massages so I'm booking one for next week. I know she knows how I feel, as the last time I went she undid two more buttons on her uniform, revealing the rose tattooed on the inside of her left breast. Her nipples were hard too, and when she bent over to wax my eyebrows I could feel them against my head. I left feeling soaking wet and had to go home and bring myself off.

Last year my husband decided he might be bi as he'd been looking at men a bit more than normal at the club. So one night he invited someone he knew was bi to the hotel we were staying at. They had full-on kissing in front of me before taking it in turns to suck each other's cocks. Then my husband asked the man to fuck him from behind, afterwards returning to kissing and cock sucking. I lay down naked beside them and they knelt on either side of me, wanking until they came, spraying all over my tits and face. We returned to the bar and drank a bottle of wine. My husband has never asked to do this again and says it was not for him. But for me it was a huge turn-on. I think watching men together is beautiful.

I often fantasise about watching my husband with other women (done it twice) and watching him have anal sex with a woman (yet to do). In my fantasies I'm truly having a bi experience rather than the odd kiss. For my favourite fantasy we go to a hotel. A girl is sitting alone – brunette, tanned, low-cut top, large but pert breasts. She smiles and I know my husband has seen her too. When he gets the next round of drinks, she turns and smiles at him and, as she turns away, he looks at me with that *how I wish* look.

I go to the loo, and she's there fixing her immaculate make-up. Suddenly I want her as badly as he does. Sensing this, she kisses me gently on the lips and asks me our room number. I tell her. Resuming our places in the bar, she smiles knowingly at me and I ask my husband if we can take the drinks back to our room. Getting a bottle of wine, we go up to 239. In the lift he immediately asks what took me so long in the loo and I explain that we were just talking, but that I'd given her our room number.

In anticipation of her visit, we pour three glasses of wine, and I change into something new that I've bought – red stockings and a small red G-string. As I dress, my husband notices that I have shaved everywhere and I can tell by the raised material in his trousers that he likes the new Hollywood look.

There's a knock at the door and I open it. It's her. I kiss her and let her in. Standing in front of the bed, she kisses me again, her hand pushing aside the material of my G-string, her fingers probing me. I stop her and tell her that first I want her to make my husband's birthday really special. She kisses him and undoes his trousers as he undoes her blouse, revealing her see-through bra, which barely contains her breasts. She pushes my husband towards the bed and asks what would make his birthday special, and he answers that it would be to have anal sex with her. She pulls out a tube of lube from her skirt and hands it to him, removing the rest of her clothes. Fully erect and needing no instruction, he goes into place behind her as she kneels on the bed over me, her head above my now-wet cunt while I get a close-up of her ass being pounded. Suddenly I feel her tongue licking my cunt at the same time. My orgasm rises and peaks, followed soon after by her ass being filled by my husband's come.

Afterwards we sit on the bed and drink wine. Then I notice his erection has returned from watching me sucking her tits in between gulps of wine. Without speaking, we both move towards his now-hard cock, licking and sucking together, our tongues sometimes meeting. As his climax approaches, I sit back and watch her finish sucking him off, taking every drop down her throat – something I've never enjoyed doing.

She asks if we'd like her to stay the night so we can have some more fun in the morning, and we agree that she should sleep in the double with my husband, and I will take the couch.

But I can hardly sleep. Just as well, since I'm disturbed by the sound of whispering. She is kneeling on the bed with her ass being filled again, her tits swinging back and forth. The look on my husband's face says it all: he is having the ultimate birthday and I know he knows I'm watching.

When we awake in the morning, we shower together. As they snog in the bedroom I appear wearing a strap-on dildo and harness. I tell my husband to kneel on the bed and, lubing him well, I enter his ass as she sucks his cock, which by now is harder than I've ever seen it. He moves towards her and enters her and we become a sandwich. Once he has filled her, she removes the dildo from me and settles between my legs and licks and sucks, then straps the dildo on and gives me a fucking until I can no longer stop the rising orgasm.

She showers and leaves. We do the same and go down for breakfast.

A Bit of Rough

Kerrigh, age 26
Heterosexual
Live-in relationship/marriage
Children
Year 12 certificate
PR Assistant
Queensland, Australia

I'm turned on by pornographic films involving a domineering man who takes the woman hostage and ravages her. Often this is in front of other men. I also love it when she's stolen and several men have sex with her. Phrases such as 'take it, baby', 'give it to me', 'fuck me, baby', 'oh, yeah, take my cock', etc., are a real turn-on. My eternal fantasy is to be that someone. My fantasies usually always start out with some domineering man taking control of my life. He might get slightly violent with me, but never excessively so. He's always passionately and erotically sorry afterwards. Somewhere along the line he shows me his sensitive side and declares his undying love, but it always reverts back to the domineering persona in which I have no choice but to give in to his needs and to my own passion.

Deanne, age 50
Heterosexual
Live-in relationship/marriage
Higher education A level equivalent
Project Administrator
Surrey, UK

I had been sexually active for four years before I got married, which lasted for fifteen years. I'd never enjoyed sex or had an orgasm. It has only been with my partner of sixteen years that I realised how great sex can be. I have sex about four times a week and each session can last up to four hours, and I have multiple orgasms. It is the greatest experience of my life.

I have fantasies about being submissive, but I don't have the courage to give my partner full control to dominate me completely. In my fantasy I meet a handsome man my age at a party and, after a few dates, we go back to his place one night. After some kisses, things start to get heavy. It's as if he can read my mind about every fantasy I've ever had but didn't have the courage to do – from being dominated by him and having no say in it, including being tied up and engaging in every possible sex act, to using toys and being spanked. With him dominating me I can let my inhibitions go and live out my fantasy.

Name withheld, 30-something
Heterosexual
Single, moderately sexually active
No children
Master's degree
Occupation unknown
London, UK

In my favourite fantasy I am dressed in nothing but a corset – one of those ornate Victorian ones, all silk-satin and lace and dyed in muted jewel tones. I've been told I'd look wonderful in a corset, so it fits in perfectly with my scenario. I'm on the bed, bent forwards onto my knees and elbows, my head bowed, forehead resting on the pillow. My wrists are bound in bondage tape, as are my ankles. My knees are kept slightly parted, my arms stretched above my head, hands resting on the pillow. A cloth of black silk covers my eyes and is knotted behind my head. The cool air kisses the lips of my cunt and I can feel it opening like a mouth, wet, ready, wanting. But that is not to be, for instead it's another mouth that will be attended to.

He moves in behind me and begins to tease me with his tongue, flicking it around and around, then darting it inside, tasting me, tasting the forbidden. He tells me how good it is, but he can't bear to wait much longer for his prize. He shifts position and I can feel the dripping head of his cock pressing hotly against the opening of my bum. I've always wanted to be penetrated here, fully penetrated, not just played with. He gets me moistened with his own juices, then pulls away. He begins with one finger, teasing, pushing in past the tight ring of muscle, then withdrawing. Next it's two fingers, he's prepping me, trying to open me up so that I can take his cock inside me. He doesn't want to hurt me; he's said so many times – that this should cause me as little pain and discomfort as possible – though we're both aware that, yes, it will hurt to some degree. My breaths are coming faster as the sensory perceptions of sight and touch have been taken away by my bondage, and he has full control over my body – and *me*. I've always wanted this, to have a man I'm really into control me like this, to have that kind of trust in a man, knowing he's only for me and I'm only for him – that it's just the two of us in this world, free to indulge any whim, any passion. (Sex, no matter what kind, should be spiritual, special, not a recreational sport. I want a man who feels like this, and *he* feels like this.)

His two fingers are lodged way up inside me, so deeply that I think they're going to tear something. But they don't. He asks me if I'm ready and I gasp that I am. I hear the sound of plastic being torn, he's putting on a condom. I don't care if we go bareback, I'd happily take a risk with him, but I don't think I want to deal with the obvious unpleasantries of what will happen once he comes inside me. He moves his cock back into place, we are dispensing with lube, since the condom is nice and lubricated anyway, and, fortunately for me, he's fairly slender in width. I should be able to take it. I hope.

And I do. I feel him sliding in, slowly, gently, little by little, more and more, coveting this place that no man has ever fully taken possession of before. To my amazement it isn't hurting, not really, and I'm so turned on by being bound, of having my backside at his complete control – Christ, he could really hurt me if he wants, injure me, and the thought excites me even though I trust him and know he won't hurt me, ever, that he will stop the moment I ask him to. But I don't ask. I push back against him, wanting the full length of him inside me, claiming me as his. All his. I feel a stretching, a fullness, it's weird, but not unpleasant, not really painful at all. (Thank God I found a lover with smaller equipment – I don't want to have sex with a donkey!) Soon he stops, and I feel his pubic hair tickling the stretching mouth of my anus; he's inside me, all the way, to the hilt as they say. I stop breathing. I'm not sure what is supposed to happen next. Neither is he. We wait. Then it's like someone has sounded a bell and suddenly I hear him breathing hard, and he starts pumping, slowly, but, yeah, he's pumping, pumping my ass, gently, then when I don't protest, less gently, and soon he's pounding into me with long deep strokes. He reaches a hand up between my thighs to find my clit and starts playing with it, manipulating it back and forth, quickly, since he knows I need a lot of steady stimula-tion to come, exerting just the right amount of pressure, his finger placed just so, not too far down or up, left or right, but right there on the location I've so often shown him (oh, in an ideal world!). He's a good student; it took a while for him to learn what works for me, but love and desire made him want to make the effort. He's playing with me and fucking me in the ass and I can't believe what's happening and I can't see, can't move my hands or my feet. I am trapped, so trapped, and I love it so much that if I died right now it would be OK. He starts to groan and I feel myself moving higher and higher and finally I am coming too, coming harder than I've ever come, with his sweet lovely cock buried deep in me, and his finger spinning my clit till I'm dizzy as he slams into me one last time, falling onto my back and sighing my name. I collapse onto his hand, blind, his cock pulsing inside me. His lovely sweet cock that I so love to taste, to suck. And now, to have inside my ass.

Cherie, age 38
Heterosexual
Live-in relationship/marriage
Children
Master's degree
Construction (professional level)
Nevada, USA

At fifteen when I discovered sex, I had been introduced to anal sex and sex during menstruation right away. I thought I'd done a lot and was fairly happy. Today I miss the fact that I didn't dare to be even more adventurous in trying BDSM (spanking in particular) or D/s games earlier. The subtle dominance in the spoken words of someone turns me on. I like people who are not ashamed of whatever kink and just being ready to do it, whatever it is. I love very tender moments in the post-sexual frenzy. I want people who don't back down from whatever they planned on doing.

I've always driven fast, way above the speed limit (by 10–15 miles per hour), and I fantasise about being arrested by a strapping police officer who would not let me go free with a ticket, but instead would play sexually with me on the side of the mostly deserted road. He would seriously spank me for my behaviour before taking his pleasure with my body and letting me come.

Name withheld, age 26
Bisexual
Live-in relationship/marriage
Some college
Self-employed
Florida, USA

I'm turned on by people who are comfortable and confident in their sexuality, those who have patience and humour and a sense of adventure, and who can see the absurdity in sex and don't mind the occasional awkwardness, people who are relaxed with themselves and make no apologies for liking what they like, people who are willing to open themselves up to new experiences and new sensations, and who aren't afraid of making a mistake.

I've always approached sex as more of a benefit and spice to a relationship than being the be-all and end-all, so what I look for in sexual partners is what I would look for in a relationship: kindness, humour, confidence, comfort and a decidedly creative mind. I want someone who isn't jaded, and can occasionally lose all sense of control, pulling me into the nearest private corner for a quickie and feel absolutely no shame from it.

My fantasies usually contain light to moderate BDSM, unusual locations, encounters that are more laughter and teasing than serious. In my fantasy I want to be put up against a wall! And I'd love to just spend a day or three naked, going about my daily routine without ever knowing exactly when I'm going to be grabbed and ravished.

Ange, age 30
Heterosexual
Virgin
College degree
Teacher
Northeast England, UK

In my fantasy I am in a darkened bedroom with only candles lit because of a blackout. A shadowed figure approaches me and speaks in gruff tones. He tells me that we are alone in the house and that I must do exactly what he says. I'm not allowed to look at him. He then proceeds to run his hands up and down my body, squeezing my breasts, while he nibbles on my neck. He begins to explain everything he is going to do to me. I will be stripped naked and fucked; if I refuse I will be spanked. I, of course, say no, at which point a sharp spank to my thigh is applied. I gasp aloud and try to turn around; another spank is then laid on my thigh again. I feel his hand running over the hot flesh which his hand has just marked. His hand then goes further up my pyjama shorts and under my knickers. He begins to feel my cunt and laughs, making remarks about how wet and how turned on I am. His fingers are rough and I try not to react to them, but I begin to move in time to the thrust of his fingers, all the while whimpering. He withdraws his hand and takes tight hold of my hips so that I can't move them. He again whispers how he is going to strip me naked and how he can't wait to see my ripe bottom. He begins to feel it as he speaks. After a short while I realise he has removed my pyjama shorts and my underwear in one go. I am naked from the waist down. I try to bring my hands up to cover myself but he holds me fast with one hand while he explores again with the other, getting rougher and rougher each time, circling my clit while, maddeningly, not touching it. I am whimpering and begging for him to touch it. He squeezes it between his thumb and fingers. I begin bucking against him while trying to get him to do it again. It is too much and his hand withdraws. He moves my legs further apart and brings me into contact with the hard bulge between his legs. He begins to dry hump me, riding against my bottom while holding me still. He pushes me towards the wall. He makes me rest my head on my crossed arms and proceeds to manipulate my body until my bottom is presented for his liking. He is still rubbing it and I am moving into the caresses.

He has rough calloused palms as if he has a job where he works with his hands.

As I begin to get bolder and move into his caresses, he spanks my bottom hard! I gasp and he hits me again and again until my whole bottom is slightly pink. He tells me it is for my own good, that I am too free with myself and that I should be punished. When he is satisfied that I have learned my lesson, he begins to pet my bottom; all the while I'm mewling with the sensation of my hot bottom, though his touch is soothing. Suddenly I feel something wet as he places a kiss there. He spreads my legs a little wider and begins to lick and kiss all of my bottom as well as plunging into my cunt. I begin to come and so he tongues me harder, licking my clit as if it's a fast-melting ice cream. He rolls his tongue and begins to use it like a penis and plunges in hard and deep. I am coming – yelling at him to do it more and harder. He quickly stands up and pushes my legs as far apart as they can go and plunges his penis into me hard and fast. He is like a piston and I have another orgasm just from first contact. He tries to prolong his own orgasm by slowing down. He withdraws almost all of him while just leaving the tip inside me. I beg him for more and he thrusts in right up to the hilt, all the while telling me what a slut I am and how wet I am for him. He pulls almost all the way out and begins to lightly spank me again with both hands on my bottom. I begin to come and this time he comes with me. We stand like that for a few moments, then he carries me off to bed and lays me down. When I awake in the morning I am unsure as to whether it was a dream or not. However, when I swing my legs around to sit up, my bottom hurts and, when I look in the mirror, I can see handprints on it. In my lipstick written on the mirror are the words 'till the next blackout'!

Kerryn, age 36
Bisexual
Single, moderately sexually active
Children
Postgraduate student
Mother/Writer/Library Assistant
New South Wales, Australia

I'm turned on by a variety of different things and situations. I like to look at the Williams Street prostitutes (in Sydney, Australia), the ones who don't look like junkies. I love a woman in knee-high boots and a short skirt ... it's the boots that do it for me. A man looking boyish turns me on no end; I love a clean-cut man with that 'private schoolboy' look: clean-shaven, short-cut hair, polite, tight T-shirt, nice jeans, big brown puppy-dog eyes. I'm turned on by the idea of going to a brothel – of women – and having sex with one or several women. Threesomes with both men and women especially appeal too.

I enjoy fantasising about forced (consensual) sex, up against the wall in a public place (but not too public – maybe a dark alley). I also enjoy fantasising about passionate, hot, long, romantic and erotic sex with the guy I've met online but never met in person! *Sigh*. We've been 'talking' online for seven years now ... I think about him in my sexual fantasies often. It's about the *passion*. This is a general idea of *one* of my fantasies: being forced to have sex or being involved in sexual activities – not rape – but enjoying being told to 'spread your legs, bitch' or 'fuck me harder' etc., etc. I like the idea of being thrown (not so as to hurt) up against a wall, roughly handled (but enjoying it), legs forced apart (of course I help a little), his hands plunging down into my pants and in my bra. It's rough but it's hot, it's quick but it's satisfying, it's horny and passionate!

Hayley, age 24
Heterosexual
Live-in relationship/marriage
No children
Further education
Carer
Yorkshire, UK

In my fantasy I get caught flirting with another person and I get taken home, where I get shouted at. The next thing I know I'm being punished by spanking; he grabs me and throws me over his knee like I'm made of air. He smacks me hard a few times but then it becomes more gentle as he starts to caress and fondle me. He turns me over and throws me down on the floor and tells me to go to my room and lie on the bed. When I get there he is close behind me and upon me almost instantly, kissing my neck and face. It gets more and more passionate until he can't take it any more and rips my clothes off; every last bit is torn in two and unwearable again. Once I'm naked, he takes his clothes off as quickly as possible and enters me and just goes for it, no pleasantries, not real foreplay, he just screws me until we're both coming. As he comes he bites down on my neck and chest, marking his territory as his and his alone. Once he is done he leaves me to think about how naughty I was.

Name withheld, age 28
Heterosexual
Live-in relationship/marriage
Bachelor's degree
Arts
London, UK

I don't mind sex being represented in pretty much any form – live and let live! But I'm worried about the lack of variety. Sex is everywhere these days, mostly used to sell things, but it's a very monochrome 'Jordan' kind of sexiness. Tan, tits, teeth! I worry about young girls learning their sexuality from popular culture this way, mostly because it might limit their imagination and make their sex lives unsatisfying and predictable. I also think it paints men in a too simplistic light. They aren't all the same, there's as much variety of taste, fantasy, etc., among men as there is among women, in my experience.

When I first started having sexual fantasies, I was very young and I was too embarrassed to fantasise about myself in a sexual situation. As soon as I saw my own face, I would feel guilty and horrible. So, to start with, all my fantasies were about other women. It was only when I got used to the idea of fantasising about myself that men started to get involved. Consequently, other women are still a big part of my fantasy life, but in practice I'm very hetero.

I'm a very controlled person in real life, and a worrier, so my fantasies tend to revolve around letting go and giving complete control to someone else. It's very much my decision to surrender that power though; I don't get turned on by the idea of being forced to do something against my will. The taboo, whatever it might be, is a very big turn-on. These days you have to go quite far to feel genuinely naughty. So, for me, that's anal sex, or maybe a rape scenario but not a nasty one. In my head it's an attractive guy that I'd actually quite like to have sex with, getting so turned on by me and my flirting, that he completely loses control and takes me, not quite against my will. Incest, too, that's a major theme. I've always been so turned on by the idea of my big brother (I don't have any brothers which probably helps!) sneaking into my room at night, perhaps just touching me at first, but over a few nights progressing to the point where we're having full sex. But the dynamic is still very brother/sister, he's telling me that he's helping me learn important things about sex and that it's healthy for a girl my age to come every day and he's the best and safest person to take care of that for me. In fact, when my boyfriend is making me come with his hand, I'm often imagining that he's my brother and running that dialogue through in my head.

I have lots of fantasies where I'm quite passive, perhaps pretending to be asleep, and someone else is taking advantage of me, trying to take my clothes off, touch me, etc. Cameras feature quite a lot, too. I love those gonzo films (haven't seen many, but enough to get the idea!) where a quite charming, likeable and attractive guy approaches random women and persuades them (with charm, money or anything else) to start taking their clothes off or put on some kind of sexual display so he can film it or take pictures for his own amusement. For me, it's the persuasion that's the sexy bit; it's about watching a woman gradually loosen up from being perhaps a bit prim at the start, to being completely slutty and up-for-it by the end. Quite sleazy, I know, but there you go!

Pregnancy is a turn-on; I guess it's quite an animal, instinctive thing. For me, as I get more and more turned on, I get more excited by the idea of getting pregnant. I don't like the feel of a cock through a condom, I like to feel it bare, to feel the come inside me and feel it coming out and soaking my pants the next day. Partly the excitement is about getting the guy to that point where he's so desperate for your pussy that he'll risk raising your kids for eighteen years just to come in it! And partly it's about the risk I'm taking myself, possibly tying myself into a relationship for the rest of my life just to get off exactly the way I like!

Cheating – my boyfriend and I share this one. I fantasise

about him creating a profile for me on some dating website, advertising me, listing all the things that I like and what I'm looking for (no-strings sex, big cock, likes deep penetration, dressed to please, etc.) and us taking really explicit pictures to send to other men. I'd then arrange to have the one with the best-looking body and biggest cock come round and fuck me while my boyfriend was away on business. As soon as he got back, I'd confess everything. I'd be all dressed up the way he likes, and I'd make him sit there, not allowed to touch me and nursing a huge erection while I told him every slutty detail of how appallingly I'd behaved, how big and hard the other guy's cock was, how much I loved it. Eventually he'd be overcome and would have to take me really roughly, bare, of course, to claim me back.

At the moment it almost feels like the naughtiest thing a young, career-orientated woman (who wants to be taken seriously) can do is to act like a Tammy Wynette-style domesticated sex slave! And although I would hate it if my boyfriend genuinely related to me on that level, I still get an erotic kick out of playing up to it (with some extreme submission thrown in). So lots of my fantasies right now go something like this: I'm at home, dressed up in a super-feminine and extremely revealing way (stockings, crippling heels, lots of make-up, painted nails, tiny leather skirt, see-through top, etc.) and I've got a list of chores I have to do, cleaning, etc. Most of them are almost impossible to achieve dressed up the way I am.

While I'm working, my boyfriend comes home, so I have to take some time out to see to his immediate needs – maybe pouring him a beer and perching on his lap as he tells me all the terribly hard things he's had to deal with that day. He'll then pat me on the bottom and suggest that I get on with my chores while he watches, relaxing in a chair. Of course, he can't leave me alone for long. He might be tempted to make things a little more difficult for me, maybe make me change my shoes so they're even higher and more difficult to work in, or blindfold me, or pull my knickers down and tie them tight around my knees so I'm hobbling everywhere. Then, after a while, he'll probably want some attention paid to him, maybe he'll require me to suck his cock for a bit or let him stick his tongue down my throat while he plays with my breasts or strokes my legs.

Eventually he'll make me stand with my back to the wall, press up close against me and stroke my pussy with my hand to make me come. He'll tell me that this was so I'll be ready to take his bare cock later on, when he feels like it. After I come, he'll leave me to get on with my work alone for a while, perhaps with a few more clothes off and with a butt plug in just to keep me ticking over.

After a while he'll come back, pull up my skirt and slip inside me without saying a word. As he fucks me, he might start to say things like, 'There's my slut, that's what you want isn't it? That's what you need, you've been so good, you deserve my cock.'

Lynne, age 31
Heterosexual
Live-in relationship/marriage
No children
College degree
Homemaker
Perth, Australia

I'm turned on by fulfilling relationships that experiment and grow together. Books play a big part and toys, plus different places where you have to plan and anticipate. My fantasy goes like this: he dribbled some oil across his hands and rubbed them slowly together. He reached out and brushed his fingers across the top of her breasts, leaving a glistening sheen. She shivered with sensation; nothing this light had left her so aware of her own body. He pushed her bra straps off and started to massage her shoulders. Her head rocked back against his shoulder, leaving her neck vulnerable. He lowered his head and nibbled. The light pain made her jump.

His hands had moved down to the top of her bra, playing around the edge. She was going to go crazy if he kept up this slow approach, she was ready to explode now. Trying to get some control back, she slipped her hand behind her and reached down to feel him.

He stood up quickly and slithered onto the bed with a determined look. 'Oh no, you're not taking control, this is my time to play,' he said, looking around the room. 'If I can't trust you to lie back and enjoy, I'll have to give you your control back.'

He had found some belts in the wardrobe and brought them to the bed and proceeded to turn her over onto her knees. She had thought he was going to tie her up, but was now thoroughly confused.

A whoosh from behind her was her only warning before her bottom was on fire. She screamed in outrage and shock. 'What the hell do you think you are doing?' she yelled at him.

Another stroke exploded on her arse.

'Be silent and it will stop,' he commanded.

'Not bloody . . .' as he administered another stroke. He waited a minute in silence to see what she decided to do. The only sound in the room was her harsh breathing as she tried to control her pain.

He poured some more oil onto his hands and massaged her arse and down her thighs. He unhooked her bra and massaged up her back, slowly soothing any tense muscles until she relaxed again. As he leaned forwards to play with her breasts, she felt his arousal brushing her bottom. Her pussy was sopping wet and he had only been playing with her for five minutes.

She rotated her bottom against his penis, trying to encourage him closer. He immediately let go of her and, *whoosh*, another blow struck her.

'I thought you were more intelligent than this? Do not move unless I tell you to.'

He returned to his playing. She didn't know what to do; her body was on fire, but she'd never let anyone take control like this. His fingers were magic, flicking her nipples, tweaking them until they were hard nubs. All her attention was focused on the sensation he was creating. He nipped her hard and she flinched away, but his tongue soothed the pain, leaving a warm glow. Over and over again he nipped, then soothed until she thought she would go insane.

Finally he moved down her body, nibbling as he went. His tongue swirled in her belly button, making her shiver. He moved behind her. He pulled her up to lean back against him, his hands kneading her sensitised breasts. His knees pushed her legs wider until she could stretch no more. His fingers brushed her curls. She wanted to push her pussy into his hands and force him inside, but was afraid of the consequences.

'Good girl,' he murmured in her ear as if he could read her mind.

His fingers thrust into her suddenly, almost lifting her off the bed with the force. She came instantaneously, collapsing against him.

'Did I say you could come?' he asked, abruptly withdrawing his fingers. She shook her head weakly. 'You're not allowed to come until I say you can. Sarah, you need to learn some discipline. I will decide your punishment later.'

His fingers were back playing in her pussy, spreading her lips and rubbing her clit lightly. He moved away from the bed.

'I want you to start playing with yourself.'

She tentatively rubbed her hands over her body, tweaking her nipples with one hand and the other buried deep inside herself. She was so glad to have control over her body again, she could feel an orgasm approaching. She started thrusting her fingers harder and deeper, with her thumb waiting to rub her clit and push her over. She had forgotten where she was, so aware of her body and its approaching climax. She heard a snap and then pain exploded on her already tender arse. She immediately stopped.

'I told you, not unless I let you,' his voice came from behind her.

She looked over her shoulder to see where he was, but the day had disappeared and all she could see were shadows.

'Don't stop touching yourself,' came another demand. Her body was so eager to come that she knew the slightest touch would send her over. She moved her hands to her thighs, slowly massaging them to try and ease the ache and calm her body down.

She heard a door open and looked over her shoulder again. He had switched on a lamp next to his wardrobe. She caught her reflection in the mirror; her bottom was striped with bright-red welts and her body undulated in time with her massaging hands.

Hands moved her around so she could see the image more clearly. They moved over her hands, slowly stretching them forwards, making her bend over.

Her bottom was thrust up into the air, displaying her to the world. Her pussy was pink and shining with her come, her butt cheeks open, and she could see her arsehole. The image was startling. She'd never seen herself like this, all flushed with arousal and on display for the world to see.

'Do you like what you see?' he whispered in her ear. 'Those red stripes really add to your gorgeous bottom.'

His hands started moulding her butt cheeks, massaging and kneading them. 'Do you like the warm feeling of the stripes? I'm going to fuck you in your arse. The first thing I noticed about you was this lovely bottom of yours. I knew then that I would see you like this with my marks on you, waiting for me to do anything I wanted.'

She was barely conscious of his words; all her attention was on the image in the mirror and the feeling it was creating.

'Have you ever been fucked up your bottom?'

She shook her head, scared of what was about to happen; she had heard that it hurt.

'It's delicious,' he continued. 'I won't need any lubricant as you have provided plenty for me. I'll slide my finger inside your arse and, while my cock is deep in your pussy, you will feel stretched, wondering whether you can take me in, but slowly your muscles will relax and I will be deep inside. I will then fuck you senseless until you beg me to let you come, and then I will finally let you.'

The images he created made her head reel.

'I do not beg,' she managed to creak from a dry mouth.

'We'll see,' was the only reply that she got.

He moved behind her again, his cock slipping around, teasing her. He slowly filled her, stopping about halfway in, slowly rocking back and forth. His fingers were oiling her arse-hole with her juices, tickling the puckered rose, making it twitch. She could see everything in the mirror, his slowly thrusting body, his cock sliding in and out, his fingers playing in her arse. She was going insane and he had only just got started.

Everything was so gentle, teasing her, putting her on edge, slowly building to the climax but never coming close to finishing. His finger slipped past her sphincter without any resistance. Everything was moving in tandem, fingers and cock, rocking slowly back and forth. A second finger entered her arse, stretching her. The movement stayed the same, and the muscles slowly relaxing let her enjoy the dark feeling this was creating.

She could feel her orgasm starting to build. His cock pulled out, but his fingers kept up their rhythm. The feeling from her bum was indescribable. She couldn't believe she was here with fingers thrusting in her bum and her dying to come.

'I'm going to fuck you now. Are you ready to beg yet?' he goaded. She shook her head, biting her lips to keep quiet.

His fingers eased out and she could feel his tip pressing gently but insistently. His fingers massaged her mound and around her clit, distracting her. She wiggled her bum and he pushed past any resistance. He paused as her body became acclimated to the new invasion.

His fingers were increasing the pressure on her clit, and she had to move in time with the motion. He started rocking, slowly easing himself in. The image in the mirror was incredible. He looked across and met her eyes and, with the last thrust, he was in to the hilt.

She was panting away, her faced flushed, but she couldn't tear her eyes away from his. He pulled all the way out and thrust deeper. Her panting increased. He removed his hands from her clit. All she could feel was his cock deep inside her bum. It was mind-numbing; she was so close to coming but couldn't.

She was out of her mind.

He continued the slow deep thrusting, slowly increasing the speed.

Then he stopped. 'Are you ready yet?' he asked.

All she could see were his eyes. 'Fuck me!' she ordered.

'No.'

As she tried to move, his hand slapped her bum with him deep inside. She flinched. The pain felt good, she was nearly there, one more thrust and slap and she would explode.

He withdrew completely and waited.

She couldn't resist, she had to have him inside her now. 'Please, fuck me, I beg you!'

His eyes lit up with savage triumph.

He plunged his cock in hard, once, twice and she exploded. He slowed down his thrusting, waiting for her to finish.

'Again!'

He started thrusting slowly, then with ever-increasing speed and hardness. Her clit was being rubbed in time with his thrusts.

She couldn't believe it, she'd just had the biggest climax ever and her body was building for another one.

'Come for me, Sarah!' he commanded and she did.

They collapsed together on the bed, spent, his cock still up her bum. He held her close, waiting for them to recover. He was still semi-erect and knew it wouldn't take much to revive him.

Sarah didn't know what she had got herself into, but she needed to recover and sleep before she learned her next lesson.

4

The Danger Zone

'Lust's passion will be served; it demands, it militates, it tyrannises.'

– Marquis de Sade

Sometimes we dream what others tell us we should not. We have chosen to explore the edge, and we have discovered that it isn't enough. The thrill of peering over the cliff no longer appeals and something inside us urges us onwards, to see and experience what is beyond that final barrier. It is here where we close our eyes one last time and dream – not of the known, the safe and secure, but of the other things, darker things, the kind of things we often can't return from. This is when we dare to fantasise just what it would be like to be in the danger zone.

This section is for those fearless risk takers willing to go wherever their desires take them. We have situations where anything can happen (and does), where things can and do get dirty, dangerous and maybe even deadly. Not surprisingly, there's a much heavier emphasis here on BDSM, bringing with it more emphasis on kink, often without a clear demarcation of free will or where the lines have blurred considerably. We see more use of control, going beyond light experimentation and play into something deeper, darker, rougher, and occasionally sinister and life-threatening. Some of the participants have already made dramatic sexual lifestyle choices, with these choices translating into their fantasies. Additional themes dealt with here include swinging, orgies and gang-bangs, shifts in gender identity, control and enslavement, rape, humiliation and death. Although there are overlaps in theme with some of the fantasies in previous sections, it is the matter of degree which places them within the danger zone. These are fantasies that frequently go to the extreme – sometimes playfully and sometimes not. There's no vanilla here, but there is every other flavour imaginable ... and indeed, *unimaginable*. For many, this is truly the point of no return.

The More, the Merrier

Leuny, age 45
Heterosexual
Live-in relationship/marriage
Children
LBO
Order Reader
The Netherlands

I've discovered that I love to have fantasies. I have learned to listen to my own body and mind and know that someday I'll have my fantasy, which is to have sex with two men. But in my favourite fantasy, I get to live in a harem and have sex with men from different countries, especially those from the Middle East.

Sarah, age 27
Heterosexual
Live-in relationship/marriage
No children
GCSE
Ambulance Dispatcher
Essex, UK

I read a lot of erotica when I was younger, but it was always the stories about sex with a stranger that turned me on. My boyfriend is a huge turn-on for me now – which is something I've never experienced before and probably sounds quite tame! I fantasise about different sexual experiences with him on a regular basis and I fantasise about actually making some of those fantasies become real. I'm probably a lot more conservative now than when I first started fantasising. I used to fantasise about lots of different men, whereas now my boyfriend tends to be the subject of my fantasies. More variety would improve my sex life. Since moving in with my boyfriend, sex has become less frequent and more predictable – still no less enjoyable, but I'd like to get a little bit more fun back into it.

One of my favourite fantasies is where my boyfriend takes me somewhere with one man or a small group of men he knows. He wants to watch each of them having sex with me in a variety of different ways until eventually he has sex with me, giving me an incredible orgasm. While each of the men has sex with me, the others attend to me, keeping me turned on and begging for more.

Name withheld, age 50
Heterosexual
Live-in relationship/marriage

Children
Postgraduate Degree and Solicitor's professional qualification
Lawyer
Yorkshire, UK

The media and society in general need to come to appreciate the sexuality and sexiness of older women, rather than focusing always on very young women or celebrities (often airbrushed or nipped and tucked, making most 'ordinary' women feel inadequate because it's nigh on impossible to get to look like them!).

For years my favourite fantasy has been to be the Roman Empress, Messalina, and to line up the whole Roman army (or at least the tastiest legionnaires) and have them one at a time, but in quick succession – perhaps in contest with a well-known town prostitute, as Messalina did. However, the idea of having one ready male after another – so if one's not that good, never mind, another is coming up – appeals most. I have a massive libido, once aroused, and the thought of being able to slake it ad infinitum with a ready supply of men who are ruled by me is very gratifying. Also, such a fantasy is totally about my pleasure, not theirs.

Tina, age 31
Bisexual
Live-in relationship/marriage
No children
Some college
Offce Manager
Wisconsin, USA

The fact that just because I'm married to a man and looking for a girlfriend doesn't mean that I want someone to fuck. I'm really looking for a companion to help me fulfil the needs my husband doesn't meet because he's socially/romantically inept, and a man. My sex life would improve if my husband were a little less impaired. Bless his heart, I love him, but he lost his virginity way too old for a guy (26), and had a string of exactly three horrible sexual encounters by the time he met me at the age of 31 (for him). I had just left a relationship where I screwed three, four times a day, every day, and all of a sudden, I had found myself in the Sahara. I now have sex with him about once every six weeks . . . on a good streak. Fortunately, we're both busy people. Unfortunately, we never get horny at the same time. Fortunately, I'm bi and he's okay with that. Unfortunately (for me) he's not bi, and I wish he were. *C'est la vie*.

I'm currently turned on by the idea of multiple people having sex at once, but not necessarily swingers. It's a turn-on for me to have 'relationship' sex. Sex with strangers isn't really interesting to me at all, because I like to be involved on a spiritual level, have some investment in it. I usually fantasise about lesbian sex, bondage foreplay (but no humiliation), blow jobs (me giving, of course), alien sex (read some strange stories once . . . haven't quite been able to get them out of my head) and food play. Hell, I used to work in a porn shop, I've got quite the repertoire of fantasies!

I had this girlfriend for about three weeks. She was quite expressive, if not very good otherwise. I also have this ex-boyfriend that was *to die for*, drop-dead gorgeous. I know he *could* be bi, and I know my husband is *not* and, of course, the girlfriend is bi, and her husband is bi too. I have a recurring fantasy about all five of us crawling into a giant pile of fluffy pillows and going at it: me sucking my husband and ex off, getting her off, watching my ex take her husband from behind while she blows him. Just one big happy wild orgy. It would never work. The only two of us who speak civilly to each other are my husband and I.

Andrea, age 33
Bisexual
Live-in relationship/marriage
College
Office Manager
New York, USA

Other than a partial bisexual experience in high school, I was always convinced I liked only men. Then a few years ago I admitted the truth to myself and my husband, and ever since we've had a great time exploring sexual variations, including toys, porn, voyeurism, exhibitionism, and swinging/group sex. In my fantasy I'm in a room with my husband having sex. We're joined by another woman and several men. I orally pleasure all the men while the woman goes down on me. Then I go down on the woman while my husband has sex with me. Afterwards, my husband has sex with me while I pleasure the other men, and the woman plays with my husband.

Name withheld, age 27
Heterosexual
Single, occasionally sexually active
Children
High School
Charity Worker
Scotland, UK

My first experiences with sex were hard as I was sexually abused as a child, but once I learned to separate forced sex and having sex through choice, I became more turned on by strong dominant women. Yukky old men are still a major turn-off though. The changes to my sexuality/sexual imagination have been more about finding things that are fun and exciting for me, rather than what pleases men. What holds me back is the lack of blokes willing to share me with other blokes at the same time! – they all seem to think it's gay to have a threesome with me and two guys, but are all more than willing to have a two-girl one-guy type threesome.

In my fantasy a couple trying for a baby go to a fertility clinic. The woman is intimately examined by a female nurse and then a male doctor while, in another room, her husband is 'helped' to produce a sperm sample by several other nurses. The details change each time I think of this scenario, but the basics as outlined remain pretty much the same.

Name withheld, age 28
Homosexual
Celibate
Master's degree
Librarian
Arizona, USA

I'd been reading books that included sex for years – I read my parents' novels starting at about age seven. When I first started to think about sex, it was in terms of their favourite Regency romance novels – the nice ones that never went past the sweetest kisses. Of course, I realised pretty quickly that I was focused on the female half of the equation and never thought about any sort of princes or heroes – I was pretty sure that I was lesbian by fourteen, and it shortly became definite. Sad to say, the best sex I've ever had has been with my Wahl coil vibrator. I've been unwillingly celibate for several years, with a dysfunctional on-again/off-again relationship with a straight girl for several years before that. I've been curious about sex parties and sex clubs for years now, but I'd never dare go to one alone, and I haven't dated anyone who'd be interested – or anyone at all – for a long time now. What holds me back is the lack of a partner, fear of disease or disaster. I like who I am – if I were straight, I'd be someone else. It would probably be easier to find a date, though.

In my fantasy I'm watching cheesy movies with my good friend, and we're both a little bit buzzed on wine. She starts teasing me about my collection of Maria Beatty films, which she found when she babysat my dog. We roll around giggling, and she asks me if I'd like to go to a lesbian sex party with her, just as friends, just to see. I am shocked, but force myself to admit to her that I'd love to.

I *would* love to – she's adorable, taller than me, strong and fit, with short spiky blonde hair and a sweet grin made slightly mischievous by a tiny silver eyebrow ring that quirks her brow.

So we meet a week later and she drives me to the party. We're both nervous and awkward, but she's been there a few times before with an old girlfriend, and I suspect that she's a lot more experienced than I am in this sort of play – I've just fantasised. A lot. She's wearing black leather pants and a black leather bodice over silk-soft skin. I'm wearing wine-red button-fly jeans and a tight black laced shirt – the closest I have to the right kind of clothes.

We're in the party – my mind fuzzes over this part – and it's hot, in more ways than one. I have my laces pulled loose on the front of my shirt, and I can smell the salt of sweat on my friend – I haven't quite dared to look at her breasts, but I can imagine the beads of liquid resting there. We're standing in a dark corner of a room full of women watching the centre of the room where two women wearing leather and tattoos are carefully binding a third woman (she's naked of everything but a blindfold) to a smoothly finished wooden and leather frame. Their hands pause to stroke and pinch as they move, their long hair causing agonised shivers as it tickles the bound woman. There isn't much room, and the watchers are growing quiet, their eyes glinting in the faint light.

My friend draws me in front of her, pulling us both to sit down, half in shadow, but we can see the three in front of us as the two tormentors begin to stroke their victim-lover with feathers and then flog her lightly with a bundle of ribbons. 'We can see from here, and I'll keep you safe,' she murmurs in my ear, her warm breath making me shiver. I feel her glare at a woman near us who had blatantly looked me over earlier – I love that, my dear friend wants to protect me and keep me to herself.

We watch, and she begins to stroke my arms – to soothe me? No, she's fiddling a bit with my laces, and I can feel her breath on my ear, and something wet – her tongue. I tense slightly, feel her tense – and then I relax against her full breasts, feel my shoulders relax, opening me to what she's offering. She hums – purrs? – into my ear and neck and begins to stroke her hands along my arms, my sides, my breasts ... As we watch the woman in front of us beg and plead, twisting as much as she can in her bindings, begging for release, my dear friend slips her hands under my shirt, stroking, twisting my nipples, almost until it hurts. I relax against her, stroking her thighs, watching, watching, with half-slit eyes. I can see other eyes across the dim room, sometimes watching the centre, sometimes closed in ecstasy, sometimes watching me.

My shirt is unlaced, my pale breasts bared to the room, tickled and shadowed by the open sides of my shirt. I am almost oblivious to the sounds, the heat, the smells of the room; I give over all control to my dear friend. She has my jeans unbuttoned and her hand strokes my belly, my hair, and then ... All I can feel is the wet sudden heat of her hand sliding firmly, quickly through my sex. I think I gasp, she squeezes my nipples together with her other hand, my legs clench – I open my eyes as I come, watching the woman in the centre come, her tormentors' mouths on her breasts, her cunt, my dear friend's hands on my cunt, my breasts, her quick breath in my ear.

Lisa, age 41
Bisexual
Live-in relationship/marriage
Children
Vocational training
Data Entry
Idaho, USA

I've become much more open-minded to exploring my sexuality and discovering what I like or don't like. I'm more in tune with who I am and am not afraid to say what I want or don't want. I decide what I like. The best sex I ever had was playing out a fantasy with my husband. We had another man come over. I had him walk into the house, get undressed, and come into the room without making any noise. He was to slip onto the bed and go down on me while my husband and I were lying on the bed kissing and touching each other. My husband is not bi, nor has he ever indulged in bi activity, but part of my fantasy was to have him inside me while another man went down on me and licked us both. I slid down my husband's cock, facing away from him and my friend followed our instructions, licking me and my husband as I rode him. A few times my husband's cock slipped out of me and my friend actually put his mouth over it, sucking as I stroked it. My husband kept his eyes closed as I was talking to him, telling him how much of a turn-on it was to watch him get sucked off by another man. Then I slid back down on him and we continued. His part of the fantasy was to see me having sex with another man and, as he talked it out, my friend did exactly what he wanted, still not making any noise or talking to us. When it came time for my husband to reclaim me, my friend slipped off the bed, watched us for a few moments, then left quietly. Both my husband and I had never experienced anything like this, but it was the best sex either of us had ever had since we both got to play out a fantasy.

I usually fantasise about having several lovers at one time, much like a gang-bang situation but with both men and women involved. In my favourite fantasy, I'm involved in a game of blind-man's bluff in a room with about fifteen to twenty people, both men and women given the freedom to explore whomever while being blindfolded. The room is lightly lit and everyone's naked except for their blindfolds. Everyone knows going into this that they may come in contact with someone of the same sex. The host of this game soaks everyone down with oil as they enter the room. You have the opportunity to explore, touch, kiss, rub, lick, fuck, or go down on anyone you come into contact with. You can spend a maximum of fifteen minutes with your partner or explore someone else before a bell is rung and you have to move on. The object is to be able to explore everyone without having to worry about what someone will say or do if you stumble onto the same sex. Everyone is there for pure enjoyment.

Melissa, age 38
Bisexual
Live-in relationship/marriage and steady relationships, not live in
Children

College degree
Medical Insurance
Ohio, USA

In life nothing holds me back. I've managed to fulfil many fantasies to date and plan to continue. In my fantasy there's me, my boyfriend Michael, my girlfriend Lori and another friend, Rob. Both men are secured to straight-backed chairs. Both have a perfect view of Lori and me as we climb onto the bed and start undressing each other. She sucks one of my nipples into her mouth, which causes me to arch my back and grab at the back of her hair to steady myself. My hands find her nipples and lightly tug on the nipple rings, which brings a moan from her onto my already-sensitised nipple. We're both making sure the guys are getting a full view of everything.

I bring Lori up for a long kiss and then trail my tongue down her neck to her nipple while I let my fingers skim over her ribs and stomach until they reach her pussy. I slide my fingers along her slit and she's wet ... really wet, so I slide my fingers into her pussy and watch her face as she starts to fuck my fingers. I let my thumb circle her clit over and over, making sure she stays on her knees. Her body is starting to tighten with the orgasm she's about to have but I stop just before she reaches it. She gets a look to her that tells me I'm in for it. She leans into me and runs her tongue along my collar, between my tits, down to my pussy and lightly licks my clit over and over, and just when I think I'm going to go over the edge ... she stops.

Lori and I have pre-arranged a lap dance that has the guys groaning ... from the sounds coming from Rob he's far from displeased with Lori's performance. Lori and I then change places and I'm giving Rob a lap dance, so close to rubbing my pussy against his bulge it's about to burst.

Lori and I decide we've denied the guys long enough and we let them loose. Both of us stand and wait for their instructions. I have a slight fear of Rob, and Michael instructs me to give him a blow job on my knees while Lori gives Michael a hand job while fucking him in the ass with one of her favourite dildos. Rob stops me before he comes and suggests we switch partners.

Lori and Rob climb on one side of the bed while Michael and I are on the other. Michael lays me back and starts eating my pussy like he's starved. While Rob is paying attention to Lori's tits and she's rubbing his cock with both her hands, I start to finger her pussy as Michael gets a glimpse. I start to fuck Lori with my vibrator. Michael uses another of my vibrators on me while licking my clit and I am just about jump off the bed with the orgasm that hits me.

Michael really wants to use a butt plug on me and believes I'm ready for it. I lean into Lori, and she begins kissing and caressing me, helping me relax. Michael lets Rob know how nervous I am so Rob starts to caress my tits, ribcage, stomach and runs his hands alternately between my ass and pussy while the butt plug is inserted. I'm relaxed and there's no pain ... there's actual pleasure and I moan into Lori's shoulder.

Once we're all comfortable that I'm OK, Lori goes on her back and Rob gets Lori's vibrating nipple clamps to attach to her nipple rings. I'm instructed to suck and lick her nipples while Rob fucks her while using the dong at the same time. Soon, Lori is having a hard orgasm.

Again, we switch positions, but at my request. Lori and I are on our hands and knees facing each other while the guys are fucking us from behind and watching us tongue and bite each other. Her fingers find their way to my clit and mine to hers ... the guys find the sight of us getting off on each other so hot that they come ... *hard*, gripping our hips so tightly that

I cry out in both pleasure and pain. Lori and Rob aren't far behind and Michael and I can hear them groan and grunt as they come as well.

Name withheld, age 41
Bisexual
Live-in relationship/marriage
Degree
Administration
Scotland, UK

When I was a girl I used to have a recurring dream about being a doll on a conveyor belt, being 'put together' on a manufacturing line. As I progressed along the line, 'parts' were 'added' to me. I was touched and interfered with by automated hands, which didn't know or care that I was sentient. I always awoke feeling 'funny'. I realise now that this was my sexual awakening. (I should clarify that I was never interfered with in real life.) This objectification desire has stayed with me. A lot of my biggest fantasies revolve around being objectified, taken for the use of others without reference to my needs, unable to react or move away from them but inwardly being deeply aroused. In addition, I would raid my father's Mickey Spillane books; they always had one sex scene in them. I used to read them while wanking, although they were conventional sex scenes and never touched on the main subject of my fantasies. My awakening as a bisexual woman took far longer. I used to deny these feelings to myself, having grown up in a homophobic household. I looked at other women and wanted to touch them but told myself I was just being competitive. It took years and a very drunken experience with an old friend before I finally accepted that it wasn't such a bad thing to want this. I now enjoy rubber enclosure, bondage and sex play, but really, I'll give anything a whirl. Nothing is more fun than the pleasure of the unexpected.

My involvement with the BDSM scene has enabled me to live out and flesh out my fantasies. Within this environment I have been able to explore my desires safely, without revulsion or judgement. It has taken years to overcome a perception that I was a closet whore, with all the societal condemnation that implies, to understand that sexuality can be good clean dirty fun so long as the people involved are all happy to engage. My husband is not 'wired up' the same way as me and doesn't take control in a sexual situation the way I would like, although he tries. He is not terribly happy for me to explore my bisexuality nor is he keen to indulge my fantasy for multiple-partner objectification. A large part of me finds little escape but to dream and read about these things. My fantasies cause arguments and tension in my relationship; sometimes I wish I didn't have them.

This is an old fantasy I wrote about when I was bi-curious. The curiosity has since been more than satisfied!

They were at a party. There weren't many there, but those who were there were beautiful. They knew nobody but the host. They had played their 'who would you do' game but gave up, because she would gladly do all the men and he, all the women.

After a little time, a little wine, and a little small talk, he whispered quietly in her ear, 'OK, so today we are going to play a game.' Her forehead wrinkled, her mouth opened to ask, but he shut it with a kiss. 'I will only play this game if you agree to do exactly what I want without question or argument. I assure you, the prize is worth it.' The game sounded interesting. She agreed to his terms.

The dining room (for it was a house party) was empty; the music was a dull thud from the living room. She stood with him, nuzzling, but he would not engage with her. A woman entered and stood five feet from them. 'She's waiting,' he said. And she clearly was. 'Go, undress her.' She protested. He whispered urgently in her ear. 'Our game,' he reminded her. 'Do this, or leave now.' So, without looking in her eyes, she slowly undressed the blonde, exposing a rare body which was both slim and full. Only when her necklace caught in her hair was she obliged to look at the blonde. As their eyes met, the blonde winked and the undresser was flooded with relief and surprise.

The job was done and the naked blonde hopped lightly onto the dining room table, legs akimbo.

'Now lick her,' he demanded.

She found that without further eye contact she could lick this stranger. She had never brought her face so close to the damp sex of another female. With trepidation but increasing arousal, she licked. In a sexual cop-out she first licked in a soft wet line from her neck. Bravery spurred a licking trail via significant proud breasts with their hard brown nipples, past softly rounded stomach, to warm wet sweet crotch. Blondie sighed and eased comfortably. She licked. She liked. And so she licked more, bringing her hands up to help her gain access to the juices, all caution ignored. She forgot herself, giving herself to the job at hand, sinking her tongue as deep as possible, using lots of spit until her tongue was silken, rubbing, as she herself liked to be rubbed.

She barely had time to consider her audacity as her own cunt began to moisten, a measure of her excitement. Imperceptibly her body began to yearn to be filled; unconsciously she knew she wanted his familiar cock inside her.

'Stop.'

Her hair was grabbed; she was forced face down on the floor. The carpet was dank; mine host had pets. She felt like one of them. Her pussy hoped for breadth and delightful depth. 'Don't move,' she was admonished. So she trembled, her nose to the vile carpet.

To her horror, she heard the unmistakable sounds of sex. She turned her head barely. There he was, fucking that blonde. He remained clothed, only his cock emerged almost humorously to service Blondie. She sounded like a porn star, moaning like a slut. Praising him, she encouraged him to drive in. 'It's good, mmmm good, go on, go on, go on!' she shouted with increasing urgency. There on the floor, ignored loins were afire, aching to be filled, attended to.

Listening to them fuck, she humped the filthy floor as much as she dared, her finger sneakily reaching for that nub of pleasure. The warmth in her spread. She was going to...she was...she...oh God...

And with a howl Blondie came, and was spent.

But on the floor, tears. She lay, frustration tore at her and she wanted him more than ever.

Her head said 'a little tenderness, a little loving please', but all she murmured was a hoarse, 'Please *now*!'

To her grateful relief, attention came her way. 'Kneel,' he said firmly but kindly. So she knelt. He rammed his damp cock into her mouth. It was still hard, and she knew already that it tasted of Blondie. She was so relieved to have him that she serviced his cock gratefully, flicking her tongue over the head, creating a vacuum and cupping his balls. He pushed harder and harder, holding her head so she couldn't escape, raping her mouth. Her eyes watered, she feared she might not be able to breathe soon, she was afraid of his power and intoxicated by it. Finally she retched. He withdrew and quickly pushed her from her knees to all fours. From nowhere he produced a blindfold and tied it tightly around her eyes. 'What do you want?' he said. Her cunt throbbed, the first tingles of orgasm from her time on the floor still clear in her mind. All she could say was 'fuck'.

The blindfold tuned her senses. She was alert to all.

With mastery, Blondie and man undressed her quivering blindfolded body. They caressed her, they kissed her and nibbled her and they licked her until parts of her glistened. They scratched her and bit her as she writhed and moaned beneath them. Her body arched to them; she tried to kiss back, to rub against them but they pulled away. At first they were careful never to place more than two hands on her body, trying to maintain an illusion that only one man was delivering this pleasure. They didn't allow the smaller female hand or an unfamiliar kiss to betray them too easily. But, when the heat in her was too high, they allowed themselves to become more carefree. At last they allowed fingers to plunge deep into her, one, then two, then more. Her groan of gratitude was almost orgasmic in itself. And when, at the same time as her pussy was full of fingers, a cock was thrust into her mouth she realised she was deceived. But she didn't care, and stopped only for a brief second before re-submitting to the bliss.

While greedily swallowing the cock in her mouth, a second cock was slid into her. Slid with the care only a woman could muster, Blondie used her solid, satisfying strap-on to deliver pussy fulfilment. Indeed, she was so wet its considerable girth barely registered. Above this doubly filled form, Blondie and he kissed, their cocks firmly lodged in the party treat below.

The fake cock was removed; the real one took its place. The relief was real. She sighed and moved against him. The fake cock was inserted in her arse, matching the real one below stroke for stroke.

So lost was she that when a third dick materialised in her mouth she barely registered that this represented yet another addition to the party. Her new playmate was not forceful, but gentle, smaller in girth than the one she was used to, but with more length. Filled in three holes, pleasure flooded her.

To her delight, harsh hands grabbed fiercely at her tits and, oh, a gentle sucking began on her clit; how many could gather around one person? This new mouth tugged gently, made her want to come, but every time she built to climax, the flicking stopped. She strained for orgasm...

He had snuck away, left her to her pleasure. He had known she would not fail him. He went to the car to fetch the newly purchased tiny seventeenth-century etching she had so admired. He had bought it for her, this was her prize. A fuck was, after all, just a fuck.

Gender Bend

Name withheld, age 35
Heterosexual
Single, moderately sexually active
Postgraduate student
London, UK

I first had sex in order to be grown-up, but didn't feel safe with anyone (first boyfriend) or orgasm, for years. I can't be bothered with casual sex; I find it boring and pointless without a mental connection. It's much sexier being walked home by someone and kissed in a way that doesn't lead to sex. I never allowed people to walk me home in the past because I felt I had to offer sex. I didn't know you could (were 'allowed to') sleep with someone and not have sex. When it comes to my fantasies, I've dreamed about Eddie Izzard, and find Pedro Almodóvar films (thinking of *High Heels*) with ambiguous men very attractive.

In my favourite fantasy I'm with a blonde woman (no one I know), stereotypical big boobs, slim – I'm me but I feel like a man. I kiss her breasts, I'm on top, I feel her, kiss her belly. My hands are on her breasts, then I lick her cunt until she's really wet (never think about the taste, don't fancy it much really – bizarre). I move back over her and enter her body. I have a cock (I'm usually using a vibrator at this point so I'm both her – being fucked – and the person doing the fucking in my mind), and I move in her hard. It's about controlling the thrusts; they are strong and hard and I want to fuck her until she's out of her mind with pleasure.

Julian, age 27
Bisexual
Live-in relationship/marriage
College graduate
Writer
California, USA

Like most people in America, I wasn't encouraged to be a lesbian, so when I first started figuring out who I might be attracted to, it was always kind of punky, artsy, femmy or androgynous women. It took a long time to develop an aesthetic where it was OK to like butch women and learn more about how women define themselves as butch. After that period, I realised that what I liked about butch women was the tension between their feminine and masculine sides. I really identified with that tension and knew there were many masculine and feminine qualities about me. Now part of my wisdom comes from loving people that don't fit simple gender or sexuality categories and wanting sexuality to be a very creative and malleable enterprise.

I'm turned on by everything that's transgender and gender-queer, such as gender-variant features of a person's body – in particular a boy that has bigger breasts than me and a small cock, and reversing the social meaning of those features as feminine, weak, ugly, strange, retarded, etc., to make them intriguing, forbidden, and multivalent – with my (female) body doing the same things, packing my pants so it looks like I have a cock, flattening my breasts, hiding my hair inside a bowler hat. During sex, I bottom more like a boy now instead of a girl, and my boy lover bottoms more like a girl.

Being in a position or having the strength and patience to have an open or multiple-partner relationship could improve things. It might also cause a lot of grief. I think being happier, having a better job, and living with another room would honestly improve my sex life. When people are cared for, happy, and respected, they have good sex. More outdoor sex would be good without fear of police retaliation.

My fantasies generally involve power dynamics, which might be power differences, or an age difference, an expert and a disciple, gendered power dynamics, etc. So this is the main tie between most of my fantasies, but their subjects, participants, details, roles, and gender always change. They involve real power differences/force that would never be OK to do in real life. I don't want to actually have underage sex, or sex between a teacher and a student, or sex with my boss, or sex while drugged and gagged, I just want to fantasise about it. Certain role-playing is fulfilling for those things.

Right now I've been having a recurring babysitter fantasy. A teenaged dorky boy, Asian or Latino, must babysit a slightly younger teenage girl. The fantasy unravels from both character's perspectives for me! They use some excuse, such as a game, dare, or re-enactment that causes them to get involved. Sometimes the boy is shy and barely makes a move. Sometimes he eats out the teenager and makes her come for the first time.

Helen, age 38
Heterosexual
Live-in relationship/marriage
Children
Master's degree
Stay-at-home mom/Writer/Artist
Virginia, USA

The best sex I ever had was with my husband. On our first date, I took him back to my dorm room and started tearing his clothes off before the door was even closed. We spent the night on my dorm room floor, and made love seven times. I could not get enough of him. We kept rubbing against each other even after we were both too worn out for intercourse. He had the best tongue I'd ever experienced, and he was the most considerate lover I'd ever had. Years later, we had another session like that where we spent all of a Saturday morning in bed together. Towards the end of it, my husband was standing at the edge of the bed, fucking me hard as I had my first ever multiple orgasm. I must have screamed for a good fifteen minutes. When I was done, I went completely limp and so did my husband. He slumped over the top of me. At first I thought it was a joke, but then I saw his eyes had glazed over and I started screaming again when he wouldn't respond to me. God, I thought I'd killed him. Turns out he had just passed out from all the exertion. We spent the rest of the day in the emergency room explaining what had happened.

I regularly fantasise about sexually dominating a younger man, someone who wants to be sexually dominated and enjoys being on the receiving end of anal sex. I also fantasise about two men having sex with each other. I married a young-looking man – though he's only two years younger than me, he's still got a baby face – so I suppose I've always had a thing for young guys. I'm nearing forty and I find myself looking more and more at men in their twenties and even as young as eighteen. I don't know what it is about younger men, but the sight of a half-dressed or nude young man immediately sends a jolt of electricity through me. I'm not talking tall muscular studs either. I want someone young, slim, about my height, someone that I could just eat alive. I imagine what it would be like to put a collar around this young man's neck and make him mine, to have him on his hands and knees in front of me, begging for my touch, either for pleasure or punishment. In some of these fantasies, I'm wearing a strap-on and my submissive toy-boy is eager to suck on it and then bend over while I push into him. Sometimes I fantasise that I have two young men and they make love to each other while I watch, and occasionally I fantasise that I am a man myself, making love to another man. These fantasies bring out the bad girl in me like nothing else does. For me, though, it's only a fantasy, and I fulfil it as much as I need to through writing and art. In real life, I'm very content to be in a monogamous relationship. The sex in my fantasies may be hot, but nothing beats a husband who helps around the house, cooks dinner and takes the kids off my hands at the weekends so I can catch a little extra sleep in the mornings.

Jack, age 25
Bisexual
Single, occasionally sexually active
No children
Bachelor's degree
Occupation unknown
Canada

I'm into gender-bending, whether it be cross-dressing or accentuating your actual gender through use of opposite gender conceits (i.e., the girl in the suit becoming more feminine) or roles. Gender play is lovely. I'm a member of the local BDSM community, and a certain level of skill with your swinging hand is sure to be a turn-on! The one I can't describe that really gets me is just a certain attitude that some people have, a sense of competence and mastery. I'm further developed as a lover of all things to do with the bum: anal sex, rimming, enemas, spanking and just showing it off at play parties.

My current fantasy is of a burgeoning threesome relationship, two guys and a girl, wherein the girl is fascinated by the dynamic between the two men. She's had sex with both of them, but she's never seen anal sex before watching them together, and she's never seen the bottom submit that way because, with her, he's always been the top. She's seen him masterful and in control of her orgasm, but never whimpering for his own. She decides that she wants to learn how to get him to submit to her like that.

First, she has him introduce her to anal sex, culminating in a lovely vaginal-anal double penetration. But then she turns the tables. She secretly buys a strap-on, and she starts to take control: first with fingers, which he hadn't expected and is incredibly turned on by, and then she pulls out her new toy and he's *really* impressed. She gets just the reaction she was hoping for, him giving it up to her. Later she does it with the third man as the audience. Much later, when he's had a very bad day and is in need of reassurance, she fists him while the other man holds him.

Though I occasionally switch perspectives, in my head I usually play the role of the bottom, whoever that is. So when he's introducing her to anal sex, I'm her, but when she's turning the tables, I'm *him*.

Kris, age 43
Bisexual
Live-in relationship/marriage
No children
College graduate
Business owner
California, USA

I love watching gay men have sex. Erotica is more of a turn-on now than it was before and I love talking during sex. The more vocal my partner is, the better. I think that someone who loves sex and loves flesh is also a turn-on. Someone who has sex for the sake of having sex – is not so sexy!

I think the best sex I've had so far has been during one 24-hour period when I had four different partners. One of them, a fuck buddy, had a small dick. But, believe it or not, he was the best. He could fuck for hours and he also had the best mouth and fingers. He's the only one who's ever been able to stick his fingers inside me at just the right spot, make me come and squirt at the same time. He was vocal and he loved to just fuck in every way possible. In that 24-hour period, we spent two hours together and at the end I could not walk. He had gone down on me and fingered me while just talking in between. Then, when he finally did enter me with his cock, he said, 'God, I've been dying for that.' I'll never forget that. Then he proceeded to fuck me and make me come over and over until he finally came an hour later. He was not afraid to try anything because he said he liked to see me come.

I love imagining that I'm a guy. Sometimes I like to get off thinking about having a cock and coming. Two guys working on me also gets me off – one in my pussy and the other in my mouth. I think two guys together is also very hot and I imagine watching two of them get off while I wank with them. My current favourite fantasy is about being a guy. I have a lovely, not-too-large cock and I am bi. I'm invited to a couple's house to 'service' both of them. I get to have them watch me while I make love to each of them. The guy is first. The bedroom is dimly lit, and contains a large bed that has a comfortable chair placed at the foot of it. The woman settles herself with some wine, one leg draped over the chair as she starts to finger her clit. The guy and I begin to get undressed and hunger sets in. We roughly remove each other's clothes and I push him back onto the bed. Sucking his cock is one of the most delicious things, and I love to hear him moan. His hands are in my hair and he grabs my head and fucks my face. My hard-on is so full it hurts. I rub myself and he is talking the entire time about how he likes it and how he's going to do the same to me. He finally lets me up and my cock is just rock hard. He sucks me but I stop him before I come. I find some lube and we're both soaking each other's cocks with it. Meanwhile, the woman is on her chair, breathing hard and close to coming. She's quiet, though. We end up stroking each other and coming loudly. She comes with us, also becoming quite loud. We take a break, get some wine, 'reset', and then I go after the woman. I love fucking women more than eating them, so the idea of a long drawn-out fucking session is hot. This time the guy is watching us and I get to watch him while I'm fucking the woman. I change positions often and finally come buried deep inside her. Sometimes the man joins us and fucks me in the ass while I'm fucking her from behind.

Candy, age 20
Bisexual
Virgin
Celibate
College student
California, USA

My biggest turn-ons are usually gender play, cross-dressing, bisexuality/pansexuality in others, threesomes, people who love to be submissive in BDSM and alt-porn. Those are the ones that jump out at me, at least. Although it's always been that way, I think nowadays even more so I find myself attracted to the so-called 'freaks and geeks' – anybody who is different I usually find sexually arousing. I want to do naughty things to nerds and I love the tattooed, pierced and otherwise 'odd'.

In my fantasy I dress up as a man – I bind my breasts, get into a harness and pack a hefty, realistic strap-on that has the perfect weight and balance in my hand, take time to dust on the fake five o'clock stubble, slick my hair back, put on the boxer-briefs that bulge obscenely with my fake hard-on, slacks, a shirt, a tie, and then I go down to a gay bar.

I cruise for a sexy, young, angelic twink who grabs my dick through my pants and eyes me up, so I force him back to the bathroom which, of course, is clean and just lovely (it is fantasy, after all, right?). He gets down on his knees to suck me off, but I drag him up and bend him over the sink and start to screw him in the ass. The whole time I get to watch both of us in the mirror above the sink – that's important to the fantasy, to have that extra layer of voyeurism and exhibitionism, as I get to see his facial expressions (and, of course, he is a fantastically greedy bottom – he loves getting it). It starts slow, but of course starts to get wild, and that's when some other guy comes in – a little older than my twink, dark haired – leans up against the wall and watches us. I can see his face in the mirror, catch his eye once, look back and focus on what I'm doing (my twink is absolutely involved in what's going on – his eyes are closed and he is oblivious to everything else). After a minute, dark-haired guy comes up behind me and shoves a hand down the back of my pants (somehow missing the strap-on harness), and starts to finger and probe my asshole while I give it to the twink. The sensations feel good, but it's more about being sandwiched, having that warm, tall, firm body to lean back against and tilt my head on, that is so great. He gives me more and more of his finger, one, then two, while his eyes stay glued on mine in the mirror, testing me, challenging me. The dildo hits my clit over and over again until I come, as does my twink. The dark-haired guy conveniently leaves and twinkie turns around and sees my dildo, much to my horror – but it turns out he's bisexual, and he eats me out in the toilet in an open stall, where a large group of surprisingly bi-curious gay men gather and watch voyeuristically, and get aroused themselves and start doing things to one another all around.

That's it, basically, in a nutshell.

At Your Service

Jane, age 31
Homosexual
Single, very sexually active
No children
Doctorate degree
Writer/Dominatrix
Ohio, USA

There are two very distinct fantasy themes in my erotic mind. The first is having very pretty eager young women service me and tend to my personal needs in a variety of different ways. Generally it has to do with their unbridled desire to kiss, lick and suck me until I'm finally satiated – at least for a while. The other subject that often excites me has to do with depriving insistent macho men of being able to touch me in any way. All they can do is gaze and drool as I sit in skimpy attire while primping at my dressing table. Often the men are gagged and restrained to keep them in total control. Fitting them with locked chastity devices is also a *huge* kick for me.

The fantasies listed above have become reality, as I have acquired the services of an ideal female companion, and I take advantage of the ideal situation at every opportunity. In addition, there are certain submissive men who have fallen deep under my spell. Thus I am able to intimately chastise them whenever I choose. The best part is they pay me to do it to them.

Mary, age 64
Heterosexual
Live-in relationship/marriage
No children
O levels
Freelance Writer/Editor
Lincolnshire, UK

I'm fascinated by people whose sexuality is ambiguous – people who might be bisexual, or else androgynous-looking women. I tend to be more adventurous as I get older. Nothing holds me back. I do it. In my favourite fantasy I'm beating my slave's bare buttocks while he pleads for mercy. I don't stop until he has promised to fuck me senseless.

Sherry, age 61
Heterosexual
Celibate
Live-in relationship/marriage
Children
High School diploma
Writer/Receptionist
Wisconsin, USA

My fantasies revolve around bondage, usually a slavery situation where the woman has been sold either by her father or her lover. If I'm thinking historically, it is the father who has sold her in order to finance his son's marriage. If it's contemporary, the man she loves has got her pregnant, then sells her to a man who sells black market babies from women he has enslaved to become pregnant.

In my fantasy, a young woman has been presented to her new master and he demands to see that she is, indeed, pregnant. Once he has examined her, he shows her how she will be treated in the future, beginning with a soft whipping. She is then forced to have sex with various partners. Of course she is carrying her lover's child, but in the future the identity of the child's father will be a mystery. In other words, she is a high-priced whore; for the men who come to this island do so with the knowledge that the expensive price tag is so they can be with as many women as possible over the period of a week, and it has cost them dearly. When the child is born, it is allowed to nurse with its mother just long enough to bring in her milk. In that way she can satisfy the needs of certain men who enjoy sucking on mother's milk.

Princess Spider, age 45
Bisexual
Live-in relationship/marriage
Children
Education unknown
Dominatrix/Writer
London, UK

I've always found black leather gloves and pearls fascinating, especially if accompanied by spectacles. Women were my first love; they seemed so delicious and sensitive. Men have to be rogues, women very feminine. Nowadays I love to say no and tease my prey. The only thing that would improve my sex life would be a man who could keep up with me.

Here is my fantasy: black-laced stockings, high-heeled shoes, leopard-skin print panties, a short leopard-skin print nightdress and gloves (leather). Remember, I always enhance my red lips with full gloss, for that all important seductive kiss. Surprise your man with this outfit and you will have him grovelling on his hands and knees. Be firm when wearing your outfit, take control of the situation; linger on the couch and cross your legs so slowly and he will think you're in slow motion. If he tries to kiss you, deny him access to your lips and simply ask him to wait. Instead distract him with your feet: ask him to remove your shoes and massage your feet so he sees your painted toenails and also a glimpse of your thighs. This is now your lingering stage . . . Your lover's urge to seduce you will be getting stronger, but be firm, keep him below your waist and get his blood boiling. Encourage the kissing of your feet, legs and thighs. If you smoke, get your man to light your cigarette, and fetch you a glass of wine. I usually demand that my lover strips and entice him to cook the evening meal . . . all distractions to aid with the lingering and lusting.

I often notice him glimpsing around the breakfast bar to see what he thinks is his prey. All the time he is sinking into my spider web, lulling him into erection and denial. Desire and frustration . . . sliding, his mind becomes confused. As he stands in front of me naked, I can see his flesh quiver . . . his erection growing.

I will stroke him very slowly with the wet fingertips of my glove, either wine or saliva, I rotate my finger very slowly over his manhood . . . Now you have him! At the very peak of his excitement simply send him back to the kitchen. I call him back and his vision has changed, now before him there are two women he has to please. Pulling him by a rope, his engorged balls full of eastern promise, I force him to fuck my slave girl while I cane his cute muscular ass...

Ravished

Hydy, age 26
Heterosexual
Live-in relationship/marriage
No children
Bachelor's degree
Bookseller/Editor/Writer
Idaho, USA

In my fantasy I get out of the shower and there is my school-girl costume on the bed. I put it on, and walk out of the bedroom. He grabs me, blindfolds me and leads me out to a van, where I'm tied up. We drive for quite some time to a cabin out in the middle of nowhere. He says he's going to take pictures of me to send for ransom. He then proceeds to snap photos from all directions, slowly removing my clothes and posing me more and more sexually. When he finishes, he says I am to earn my keep while I'm here, and sets up a video camera. He tells me I'm a very naughty girl, posing for naughty pictures for him, and he proceeds to spank me for the camera. Then he fingers me, finding me wet, spanks me a bit more, telling me I'm naughty and saying if I want him I should beg for it. Desperately turned on by this point, I do. I beg him to fuck me, pushing myself towards him until he does. He takes me, fucking me until we both collapse in exhaustion.

Name withheld, age 45
Heterosexual
Single, moderately sexually active
Undergraduate degree
Manager
California, USA

I've always found alpha men a big sexual turn-on. I love a man who takes control and won't take no for an answer. I still love alpha men, though now they seem to be a bit more toned down. I don't mind finding that they're vulnerable or have faults, but they still need to be alpha men. The best sex I ever had was with a man who at first was a friend: lying in bed together, learning about each other's bodies, not rushing anything, the touching and kissing, foreplay lasting for over an hour. Then, when neither of us could stand it, he filled me on the very first thrust. I love forceful men who realise that I like the build-up, but when I say 'harder' they listen and give me what I want. I'd like to find a man I can trust with my most intimate secrets and desires.

My favourite fantasy is being kidnapped by a man who wants to teach me about his sensual world. It starts off very innocently, with him teaching me how to arouse my own body and his – to full penetration, anal sex, sex with multiple partners, and eventually being involved in a relationship.

Virginia, age 56
Heterosexual
Single, moderately sexually active
No children
Bachelor's degree
Author
California, USA

I had orgasms at the age of seven. I fantasised about naked people upside down on crosses (I'm Catholic), being held naked in a cage with strangers' hands touching me through the bars. I got physically turned on while listening to my girlfriend read the novel *Candy* at fourteen. I was date-raped at twenty and loved it. I make love stoned with my ex-husband, with his wife's consent. Sometimes we do a threesome. Trust and honesty are very important. And we laugh a lot during sex. We've also discovered 'pain-gasms'. He massages me and I direct him, plus I get him to do it really hard. It makes me come. Actually, I've done most of my fantasies. But I'm always in charge, not a victim. I love masturbation these days. I'm getting picky about men and don't like to wait around for satisfaction. Wish I could find more reliable toys. The ones they make are so cheap!

I like to imagine being abducted by men and being sexually aroused with a variety of dildos until I'm begging for sex. Bondage usually enters into it. Repeated rape. People watching. Dirty words. Threats.

Shauna, age 35
Bisexual
Steady relationship, not live-in
Children
Master's degree
Psychologist
California, USA

My fantasy themes generally revolve around being tied up, spanked, nipple torture, flogging, anal sex, sex with strangers, sex in public, and sex with specific co-workers (damn, this one guy just exudes sexuality!). I think I'm more sexually sure of myself and am not afraid to ask for something that I want.

Do this, do that . . . Also, I'm more willing to try new things and to have frank discussions about sex.

I have this recurring pirate fantasy where I'm held captive by a pirate and tied to the main mast. The captain flogs me and tortures me, and then fucks me using every available hole. He lets all the other pirates use me and abuse me, and then takes me to his cabin and treats me like the lady I am, making love to me gently and lovingly. The only thing holding me back from fulfilling my fantasy is the lack of a pirate ship. Found the pirate!

Christina, age 41
Bisexual
Single, very sexually active
Children
Post-secondary education
Paramedic
British Columbia, Canada

I'm turned on by people that are kind and make me laugh. I have to admit that the sign of a large bulge in the front of a pair of tight jeans is also a big turn-on. Giving a man oral sex is an extreme turn-on for me too. I used to be very shy and very reserved. When I met my husband things were good and then after my kids left home I was just not happy. I was becoming more and more sexually frustrated and he was not interested. Now I'm single and find I am the opposite, almost to the extreme. I am *very* sexually active and just can't seem to get enough. I have also approached men directly for sex, which I would *never* have done.

I have had some tremendous sex and the size of a man's penis is not only a turn-on, it does make a difference, though I have had sex with one man who was very small and it was absolutely wonderful sex. I think one of the reasons sex with the smaller-equipped man was so good was that he spent so much time just having fun, making me laugh and he was a *marvellous* kisser and kissing is huge for me. He was also incredible at giving me oral sex to the point that intercourse was almost just a little something added on at the end. On the other hand I have had sex with big men that took time as well and the submissive feeling of submitting myself to a man that's big is intense for me. I was very well prepared by this one man, who was also a good kisser. He laid me down and moved up between my legs, which I opened willingly. He sucked on both my nipples, which was incredible, and he kissed me and looked at me and told me he was going to fuck me and come in me. The way he said that made me melt and, without waiting for a comment, he entered me slowly, but all the way, and he was very well hung. Feeling that big penis invade me and fill me was awesome. When I felt his balls pressing against me, he moved down again and kissed me fully and began slow short thrusts . . . my first orgasm was almost immediate. He picked up the pace and alternated from short to long deep strokes and talked dirty to me. The combination of all this was extremely intense, and he looked at me and told me when he was going to come inside me and that alone made me orgasm again.

I have also had sex with women. I find that to be very soft, very slow-moving and very erotic. I wouldn't say I prefer it to male/female, but it is different and it is very erotic. I enjoy kissing a woman and, while I'm more submissive with a man, I seem to be a little less so with a woman. I'm not dominant, but more equal I guess.

I have also engaged in sex with a dog. A girlfriend of mine does it all the time and I finally watched. I think it was the amount of semen that got me as I do seem to be fascinated by semen. When she finally talked me into trying it, we had been playing with each other so I was very excited and 'horny'. She helped prepare things and got me relaxed enough to try, and I thought 'what the hell', so I got on my hands and knees and she got the dog up onto me. She guided him into me; at first it felt very hard and almost sharp, poking me. When he pushed a little harder, I felt his penis swell inside me and it was shocking. As the dog began to pump, he grew in me and I was beginning to feel very excited. The thrusting only lasted a few minutes, but at one point his penis felt huge; the 'knot' near the end of his penis penetrated me, and the dog pumped like mad. The entry of that 'knot' and feeling the penis swell enormously in me did make me orgasm and, shortly after, I could feel the dog coming in me, as a dog's semen is much hotter in temperature than a man's. Feeling all that 'hot' semen being injected into me caused multiple orgasms and I was out of control. When the dog stopped pumping, he remained in me for a few minutes and I could feel the hot semen oozing out of me, and I continued to orgasm. When he withdrew, my friend collected almost half a cup of semen that ran from me. Those were the most out-of-control orgasms I have ever experienced, but I don't tell very many people about that one!

While I have several fantasies, the one I seem to think of most often is a 'mock' rape where someone I don't know (but who is safe and friends with close friends of mine) takes me out and is very dominant with me. He seduces me until I am highly aroused, then forces himself on me, tears my clothes, blindfolds me and rapes me over and over. This man is also very well-endowed. While I am actively pursuing my fantasies, the 'rape' fantasy is one I have to be very careful of because I would have to know the person and script it out first. While I dream of a stranger, I know I could never relax and enjoy that.

Name withheld, age 51
Homosexual
Live-in relationship/marriage
Some college
Drug/Alcohol counsellor
West Coast, USA

I'm turned on by watching other people 'play': whipping, flogging, fisting ... the aroma of sweaty leather, the feel of a whip ... Control and overpowerment are the themes running through my fantasies. This has grown thanks to the inclusion of sex with a twist in my BDSM lifestyle. Experience and maturity have also made a difference in the way I approach life and sex. What holds me back is the fear of enjoying it. It's a matter of trust, and the desire to have it come true. Sometimes fantasies are best kept a fantasy.

In my favourite fantasy I'm being held against my will in order to be sexually seduced by three to five women ... to get fisted, fucked and made to come until I can no longer come, totally spent ...

Love Hurts

Name withheld, age 51
Bisexual
Live-in relationship/marriage
No children
Bachelor's degree
Writer
Oregon, USA

I'm currently turned on by rape, bondage and S&M with female tops. My fantasies generally involve two males. In my favourite fantasy, one man's face is between my legs, while the other is taking him in the ass. Preferably the man getting sodomised is straight. One or both is marked by my whip. The only thing holding me back from acting out my fantasy is that I haven't found the right second male.

Marilyn, age 47
Bisexual
Live-in relationship/marriage
No children
Some college
Writer
Ohio, USA

I was always very erotically attracted to older girls who had bad attitudes, or misbehaved somehow (but not tomboys, I always liked very pretty girls), and I was always erotically turned on by ideas of discipline, humiliation, and being dominated by them. This goes back to even when I was six or seven years old, and then just continued being part of my sexual make-up forever, only it eventually included men. Any time I saw pretty older girls in movies or on TV who were at all provocative in their behaviour, I fell in love with them. Pamela Franklin in *The Prime of Miss Jean Brodie* comes to mind! I was hopelessly in love with her. But there were so many girls I had crushes on back then, and also girls in real life – I was in love with most of my babysitters and privately wished they would punish me; I fantasised about it almost constantly. Yet, in reality, I was extremely well-behaved.

I have recurring fantasies about my girlfriend, where I re-live B&D sex we've actually had together that has been really,

really great. I fantasise about being able to take time off with my girlfriend (who I don't live with, btw; I live with a man), go to Paris and stay in my other girlfriend's apartment when she isn't there (!), then just have a ton of sex with my girlfriend. In real life, she is an insatiable top, and I am an insatiable bottom. So I fantasise that we have all the time in the world to exhaust ourselves with B&D scenes (and drink wine). I don't know why I always imagine that we do this in Paris, though! Or why it has to be in my other girlfriend's apartment when she isn't home. And I imagine there are all kinds of handy sex devices in the apartment too, like slings, B&D contraptions and stuff. My other fantasies frequently involve gang-bang-type scenarios, but not really brutal. More it's about being with five or six men at once of all different physical types and races, who all instinctively know every nuance of my sexual needs and desires. There's no need for any kind of talking. The communication and sexual rapport is instantaneous. There is a lot of domination because I am submissive, but the fantasy is not about brutality, it's about satiation without having to ask for it or justify what I want.

Name withheld, age 27
Bisexual
Single, moderately sexually active
No children
Degree
Housing
Glasgow, UK

In my favourite fantasy I'm in an old wooden house. Its doors and windows are broken and unhinged, the mosquito screens torn. The paint is old and peeling. The floors are unfinished wood and there's very little furniture. What's there is old and damp and ugly: a 1970s couch and Formica kitchen table, an old iron bed in each upstairs room with a mattress and no sheets or pillows. The house is out in the middle of nowhere, and grass is growing wild on the lawn.

There are a couple of versions of this. In one, I'm stranded there with several men who talk harshly to me. There is always one man who's talking, telling the others what to do. The others are silent, except for occasional observations about how I'm reacting to what they do. I'm dragged upstairs, tied to a bed or held down. I'm whipped and scratched. One man is ordered to pinch my nipples, one is ordered to scratch my thighs, one is ordered to whip my stomach, etc. The man who's the leader forces me to come, usually with his mouth. Just before I do, someone kisses me roughly, first on the neck, then on the mouth, so that I can't breathe. Sometimes it's this same scenario, but with only one man.

Another version is more playful. I'm in the same house with several people, women and men. But this time it's like a game to see how I'll react to what they do to me. There's always one person watching, usually a man, while it's usually the women who stroke my breasts, lick me, tease my pussy with their breath. Sometimes it's like a punishment for something, but I don't know what I've done. I can hear them talking about how hard I'm going to come.

Deanna, age 33
Bisexual
Live-in relationship/marriage
Children
Bachelor's degree
Writer
Texas, USA

I never considered lesbianism as an option until college, so I was always turned on by 'hair bands' and new wave acts. Actors, celebrities and rock stars were my turn-ons then. I envisioned sex within marriage or a long-term, safe relationship. Now my husband is a turn-on. Just being with him makes me excited, sharing our lives together and our family.

I love bondage. I am fine being the submissive or the dominant. I have 'controlled' rape fantasies concerning beautiful female celebrities. I enjoy role-playing like naughty schoolgirl and hunky teacher. I also have a lot of lesbian fantasies as I'm married to a man and don't get to sample that aspect of my sexuality any more. I had that experience only once but have wanted to revisit it again and again.

In my fantasy I am in a dungeon, looking like Salma Hayek with overflowing breasts and long curly hair. I'm wearing a black leather bodice, flowing skirt with nothing underneath, and thigh-high boots. The area is dimly lit, with long black, red and white candles. There is a musky scent in the air reminiscent of patchouli. A beautiful Angelina Jolie-type woman lies on a table, naked, with her legs and arms spread apart. She is bound and gagged with red silk scarves.

I walk over to her and run my cat-o'-nine-tails along the length of her body. My husband is watching, breathlessly, in the corner. He is naked and bound to the wall. I am in complete control of the situation. I rub the whip against her breasts and *thwack, thwack, thwack* three times each. I then take my left glove off and knead her nipples, one by one, between my thumb and forefinger. She begins to moan and bites her scarf. I see the pleasure in her eyes so I bring my tongue to meet each nipple. I put them in my mouth and nibble, gently at first. I suckle her like a newborn babe and then bite down hard.

I release my grip and whack her again with the whip, this

time harder and faster. She arches her back and pushes her back down. I step away from the table and return with clamps, which I fasten to her breasts. I twist them several times. Afterwards, I run the whip down to her lower abdomen. I strike her gently. I kiss and lick around her belly button and pelvic area, avoiding (on purpose) her genitals. I'm not ready to release her yet. I knead the soft flesh there and move my hands downwards. I reach her labia and gently open the folds with my fingers. I take my fingers and explore her insides. I find her clit and move my mouth down to nibble on it. I suck on it and lick it and run my tongue all over it. She urges me onwards so I stop.

I walk over to my naked husband in the corner, whip in hand. I strike him several times on the legs and hands. I then lean forwards to suck his hard cock. I lick him from tip to testicles and back up again. I take my hand, using a tightened up-and-down grip while sucking, until a little bit of pre-come flows into my mouth.

I release him and let him enter the beauty on the table. He is fully turned on and ready for action. I walk over to the girl, stroking her hair and breasts. I remove the silk scarf and kiss her passionately. After my husband spills his seed inside her, I get on top of the table and rub my hardened clit up against her. I leave my clothes on so she can feel the texture of my skirt. I lean forwards and kiss her again, undoing her hands. My husband undoes her feet.

Then we switch positions. They both bind me and strip me naked. They take turns exploring my body, making me come over and over again with their tongues and the various implements I have in my 'pleasure chamber'.

Ariel, age 44
Live-in relationship/marriage

Heterosexual
College
Writer
Nevada, USA

I think I've always been curious about women. They look like me yet every one is different. On the other hand, I've always loved men and can't quite figure out how things would end up without a cock involved. My daydreams used to revolve around being hurt in some strange accident and saved by someone heroic (like in *Starsky & Hutch* or something) and falling into bed with my rescuer (which, having just been shot or something, seems unlikely now).

My first true sexual fantasy (other than dreaming about oral sex which I did for years before I ever imagined people did such things as 'kiss each other there') involved being kidnapped and taken to an abandoned warehouse, where people were touching me and undressing me and looking at me. I was a teenager and thought I was writing a short story. I got kind of alarmed at how it made me feel and got rid of it. But the idea of being out of control – when in real life I'm not usually – is still a distinct turn-on; it has just evolved into long, very detailed scenarios. After twenty years my husband still turns me on like anything. I love being spanked or tied up or told to do something. I love sex outdoors and don't get enough of it. I really love sucking on him and I like it when he just takes control. When I was younger before we got together (we got together when I was 24 and he was 33) I was afraid of my fantasies. I thought it was weird to be interested in women when I was clearly fucking males (randomly in college for a while), or wanting to be spanked or punished or wanting kinky things like ice or heat or having someone use a belt on me. My husband is even more open than I am and we've explored a lot of my fantasies, though even after twenty years he has to pry them out of me slowly.

My fantasy is a kind of blend of domestic discipline and BDSM. I'm with a friend and we're talking about something I've done that I'm not supposed to have done, like buying something expensive or driving too fast (we live thirty miles out of the city and drive in together every day) and, as I'm talking, I don't realise that he's behind me. She suddenly looks over my shoulder at him and I freeze because I know I'm in trouble, but I figure he'll at least wait until my company goes home. But he doesn't; he tells me to come into the bedroom with him and tells her I'll be a couple of minutes. I protest and, even with him alone in the bedroom, I'm saying, 'No, you can't be doing this now, she'll hear us.' He tells me that I wasn't so concerned about him hearing my confession and that I have mere seconds to pull my pants down and get over his knee. I don't, of course, and he finally forces me, ripping off my shorts and panties and putting me over his knee and starting to spank me very hard. I'm squirming and protesting and saying, 'Don't. She'll hear us. At least wait till she goes home so she doesn't hear,' and he says too late, and I look up and she's there. I start shouting at her to go away, but she's curious about what's going on and comes in to watch and, of course, he lets her. I'm throwing a fit by then, calling her a bitch and swearing at him and he responds by restraining me, then turning my ass bright red. I'm thrashing so hard he says he has to calm me down and he has tranquilisers that are suppositories. She asks if she can put them in and I'm calling her a bitch and everything I can think of, but he restrains me and she slides them ... slowly ... into my ass and then, with his permission, gives me some stinging slaps. She says she doesn't like what I called her and can she wash my mouth out? He says yes, and she gives me a sliver of soap and he puts me in the corner to hold it in my mouth till it's gone and to stay there. The two of them leave the room together and when they come back for me, it turns out he's decided she's going to be my caretaker whenever he's gone; I have to answer to her. She's grinning like a cat that has swallowed the whole canary.

Anniemc, age 46
Heterosexual
Celibate
Separated
Children
Associate's degree
Nurse
Ohio, USA

I enjoy fantasies about submission to a 'daddy' male – male domination/female submission themes – a take-charge man with a willing female partner. I enjoy male control of female sexuality by means of bondage, discipline or demands, with the male being committed to the female (of course!) and caring for her outside the bedroom too. The best sex I ever had was when my husband held my arms down and sucked, pinched and bit my nipples, when he forced my legs apart and spanked my pussy, when he played at being my daddy. We never went far enough with this, but I loved it when we did. He would sometimes gently fuck my face with his cock; if it got too rough and I wasn't aroused it was awful, but the few times I was turned on and he slowly thrust I loved it. I wish I could go back and tell him how much I loved these acts of sex. It's too late now. The opportunity is long past, and I now realise what I had but lost thanks to not communicating my desires to my husband. We rarely spoke of desires. We both lost out. Before we divorce (for the second time I might add) I think I will just tell him my desires. Really, what do I have to lose? Only my pride – and he isn't likely to embarrass me over my desires.

I will just ramble on with ideas that usually occur in my daydreams. I realise this is a fantasy, so these situations will likely never occur in real time. Ahh, but my heart desires . . . Anyway, I daydream about a male with power, a sound mind, strong body and universal knowledge. He sees me for what and who I am. He is accepting. He doesn't speak falsehoods about my body, but he does find things to praise about it. He overlooks cellulite, less than ideal muscle tone. He likes touching my body everywhere. He teaches me how to please him, he guides me so I learn how best to give him what he needs. His cock is large enough to fill my large pussy. He takes the time to give me orgasms (as I am slow to peak). He binds my smallish breasts so they swell. He bites, sucks, pinches, spanks, clamps my nipples. He will tease and love me with gentleness as well. Our sex is not always rough and painful. He pets, slaps, spanks, sucks, licks, bites my pussy and clit. He talks to me using crude, specific, graphic and descriptive words. He knows female sexuality is very brain-based – he exploits this knowledge to the max with me. He will at times drive my desire to a fever pitch, just to leave me pulsing with desire but without release. He takes the time to train me to take his cock down my throat, up my ass, to take a beating with a belt when needed, to take the enema he gives me, to suck off his friend if he so desires it. I learn to love and accept it all. I learn to love my tongue up his asshole. I learn to hold my orgasm until he permits me to come. I crave his touch as he craves mine. He finds joy, peace, contentment and satisfaction with me as I do with him. I don't call him Master, but at times Sir or Daddy are the names I use (depending on the situation). I think about being exposed to someone while my man is having sex with me. I think about bondage. I think about vibrators, plugs, paddles, no costumes other than bras.

Risky Business

Crystal, age 25
Bisexual
Single, moderately sexually active
Children
A levels
Student
Wales, UK

I fantasise several times a day. I like to fantasise about 'rape', bondage, restraints, humiliation and group sex (where I'm used by several men, unable to escape or stop them). I discovered BDSM about a year ago and kind of 'grew into' my sexuality. It had always been there, I'd just never known why or understood why I liked certain things (like sex with clothes on, a struggle, blindfolds, etc.). I'm turned on by people in control, filthy language when I'm aroused, dominance. I have written my fantasy as a short story.

Her breath quickened as she heard him pace around the bed where she was laid, wrists bound together and above her head, legs tied apart, one to each bedpost, and blindfolded. She could hardly move; so tight was the rope that even the slightest pull on it chafed her skin. The only way to keep it from hurting was to remain perfectly still. She had no idea how long she'd been lying there.

The footsteps paused at the foot of the bed, where her skirt had been bunched up to her knees to allow her ankles to be bound. She was acutely aware of how vulnerable she felt, not even sure whether her knickers were exposed to him. She shivered.

'Nervous?'

She jumped a little at his voice, unused to the noise; it had been silent forever. She nodded her head, knowing full well that her voice would fail her if she tried to speak.

'Thirsty?'

Again she nodded. She heard the footsteps approach her left side, heard the chink of the glass on the bedside table, and almost immediately felt the straw being pushed into the corner of her mouth. She sipped on the iced water gratefully, feeling her throat calm as the cool liquid washed over it. She nodded when she'd had enough and he removed the straw and replaced the glass.

'Thank you,' she croaked, unsure whether it was arousal or fear that cracked her voice so.

'Good girl.'

She felt something drag softly across the top of her thigh, moving down slowly to her knee, down her shin, down to her foot. She remained silent as he repeated this in reverse on the other leg, starting at her foot, up her shin, over her kneecap, up her thigh . . . she felt him encounter the hem of her skirt and she tensed up momentarily before calming herself, remembering that she trusted him. He continued tracing his finger across her skin, moving under the skirt and upwards . . .

She could hardly keep from gasping as his finger met the crease at the top of her leg, trailing the line of her black cotton underwear. Gently, so gently, he touched her through her knickers, feeling her dampness through them. He murmured his appreciation before leaning in towards her core and inhaling deeply. She baulked, suddenly feeling very helpless and exposed. He stopped dead where he was, waiting for her to relax, but she couldn't. Having someone that close was too intimate – it was way past her comfort zone. Her breathing became shallow; she would tell you it was panic but her cunt would disagree, becoming wetter and hotter with every passing second that his face remained in its proximity.

He smiled. He loved that he could still make her feel so defenceless, so ashamed, so apprehensive. He exhaled a long hot breath directly onto her pussy, making her moan involuntarily and writhe against her restraints. She hated that she wanted him this much. Hated and loved it.

Suddenly, he was gone. Disappointment coursed through her but, determined not to show it, she bit her lower lip and remained silent. Unfortunately, biting her lip was a betraying sign – he already knew how aroused she was. And how very frustrated.

Silence. She strained to hear him, but could no longer work out where he was, arousal having disorientated her senses further. From nowhere she felt the cold scratch of metal across her collarbone. She froze, half afraid and half aroused. She felt him move inside her blouse and slice upwards, heard the slash as the flimsy material tore and fell to either side of her chest, felt the cool air on her skin . . .

The knife (she assumed it was a knife, anyway) was on her skin again, playfully drawing circles across her cleavage before finally dipping inside her bra and again slicing upwards, freeing her breasts from their restraints as it fell away. She shivered, but wasn't cold. It was the blade, now resting on her erect nipple. She realised she was holding her breath.

'Are you afraid yet, little one?' he teased.

She didn't respond, knowing that any motion would jiggle the knife. She just lay there, naked from the waist up, blade at her nipple, her cunt becoming more soaked by the second. God, she needed this.

She felt the warmth of skin, his hand she thought, on her knee. The knife hadn't moved. He moved his hand upwards, dragging his fingertips along the insides of her thighs. She moaned and couldn't help rotating her hips as he approached where she needed him most.

'Now, now, slut, you know you shouldn't move while I'm holding this near to you,' he scolded, tapping the knife against her breast and removing his hand from her thigh. She whimpered. 'Would you like to try again?'

He didn't wait for an answer, just replaced both the icy metal blade to her nipple and his soft warm hand on the inside of her knee. This time he moved his hand up slowly, deliberately, and yet she remained still. He stopped millimetres from her, feeling the heat from her aching cunt already. He knew how badly she needed to come, but he wasn't about to give it away that easily. Not just yet.

Her breathing slowed as she regained control of herself. The knife vanished from her breast, leaving her free to inhale deeply. As she did so, she felt her skirt being lifted and pulled around her waist, leaving her in just her underwear. She immediately flushed with embarrassment, knowing that she was drenched and that he would now see it, too. She pulled her wrists vainly against the bonds, trying to stop him from moving himself down between her legs. He smirked and positioned himself between her thighs, face close to her crotch again. He made a show of breathing in deeply, savouring her scent as well as her shame. He knew how difficult she found this, and was slightly surprised that she'd not called *amber* yet. Still, learning not to question a good thing, he scratched the knife against the side of her now-soaked knickers.

'I think we should take these off. You've drenched them – they're not really fit to wear any more.'

She blushed scarlet, humiliated at his words and reddening further as she accepted that he was right. He sliced them away in one swift move, and pulled them from under her ass.

He threw them at her, landing them on her face, much to her shame. She tried to shake them off but the cool of the knife against the inside of her thigh stopped her in her tracks. She lay there, feeling him inches from her pussy, her drenched pants draped over her face, forced to breathe in her own scent. A tear escaped from the corner of her eye.

He extended a finger and traced the outline of her perfectly smooth pussy, waxed that day, as ordered. It was soaking.

'You really are a dirty little bitch, aren't you? This cunt is absolutely drenched. I wonder, is that because you're enjoying your own scent? The scent of your aroused, open, aching pussy? Tell me ... is it?'

'Yes, Sir.'

'Good girl.'

She sighed, desperately frustrated and highly aroused. He got up and removed the underwear from her face, moving them close to his face and breathing in deeply once more before discarding them. He lowered himself until his mouth was right by her ear and, as he started to whisper exactly how he planned to make use of her sodden cunt and hungry ass, he began touching her nipples, circling around them before kneading the whole breast. He assured her that he would make the very best use of his slut before the night was out. She whimpered again, crying now with frustration and utter lust.

'Something you want, slut?'

'Oh, God, I want you, please, fill me, please, I need you, I need something inside me ...' she begged.

He knew she was in a state – she never begged. Ever. He moved around, putting his face close to her again, making his intentions blatantly clear. She didn't even object, despite finding oral too intimate to be comfortable usually. He smiled. This is what he loved about dominance – the ability to change someone's reactions.

He leaned forwards and planted a kiss right on her clit, sucking it into his mouth gently as he slowly pushed two fingers inside her pussy. She grunted immediately and tried to push her hips up into his face, but the restraints prevented too much movement. He released her clit and started licking in long delicate strokes up and down, before returning to it and circling it softly with the flat of his tongue. He removed his fingers from her dripping cunt momentarily before jamming them brutally back inside her, adding a third, and thrusting repeatedly against her G-spot as his tongue continued licking and suckling at her clit. He could tell she was close – she'd been on the brink for what felt like hours.

Her stomach started tensing and she recognised the almost-discomfort of impending orgasm. He moved his head up and jabbed at her insides faster, furiously, until she groaned loudly and started to shake, orgasm now inevitable. With a final few thrusts he plunged his fingers deep inside her as she came so hard she actually released fluid, and moaned so loudly she even startled herself. She shuddered as he relaxed his touch, the thrusts becoming light strokes now, more to comfort than to arouse. She wept openly as he finally removed his fingers and offered them to her to clean. She licked and sucked until she could no longer taste any of herself on him. He cradled her and smoothed her hair, telling her she'd done so well coming that hard and that he was so proud of her. She settled, the tears soon replaced with words of adoration and gratitude.

'Good girl. God, I love making you come like that.'

She was rarely comfortable to let go like that; she'd gushed maybe twice in her life. She was instantly embarrassed and began to fret, but being bound there wasn't a great deal she could do about it. He climbed off her and stood at the foot of the bed again, staring right up at her.

'Oh, my God, you should see the mess you made. God, that's horny. You're fucking soaking, slut. Your thighs are drenched, your cunt is open and hungry ... I will need to fuck it soon I think.'

Even though she was still in the throes of her orgasm, she felt her cunt clench as he spoke. She had never wanted anyone quite this much.

'Oh, God ... please ...' she cried, 'Please fuck me. I need you inside me, please?'

'We are impatient, aren't we, slut?'

She felt him at her feet, her ankles, but couldn't make out what he was doing. It was only once he'd undone the second one that she realised she was free. She thanked him immediately, but should have known that it was never that simple with him.

'On your knees, fuckslut. Face on the mattress. Arse in the air.'

It was the most degrading position for her, she hated it. So exposed, so open, just ready to be used. She turned herself over, the wrist restraints being flexible enough to turn around even if they didn't let her move away much. She pulled herself up onto her knees with difficulty, knowing that he was watching and enjoying the spectacle, more so knowing how embarrassed she was. She lay, arms outstretched in front of her, face down, arse up in the air, and waited.

'Good girl,' he said finally, before she felt him touch her dripping cunt again.

To her shame, she felt moisture dribble down the insides of her thighs, and she flushed crimson knowing that he, too, could see it. He scooped some up and smeared it over her arsehole, slowly massaging her puckered hole until she was relaxed enough to accept his finger as it probed inside her. To her shame, she found herself grunting and pushing back on him.

'You dirty, filthy little bitch. You want me to fuck your arse!' he exclaimed, unable to hide the elation in his voice.

She whimpered in reply, pushing her face harder into the pillow as he continued his invasion. Finally she felt him withdraw his fingers – she wasn't sure if she was relieved or not, but she felt desperately empty. He rubbed his cock all around her drenched cunt, smearing it in her abundant juices before holding it steady at her tight opening. And then he just stopped. She moaned in frustration, but still he remained frozen. Calmly, eventually, she heard his voice.

'Beg for it, little one. Beg for your Master to use his slut's arse. Beg to come with my cock inside you. Make it convincing and I might allow you to ...'

'Oh, God, please ... I need you ... I need to come, please, please fuck my arse, Master, let me feel you inside me ...'

She was still pleading when she felt the first thrust as he plunged his cock deep inside her hot tight arse. She whimpered in pain, and then in pleasure, then in pain again; she hated not knowing whether she loved something or whether she hated it. He fucked her slowly, speeding up just when she started to panic and slowing down just when she started to come. She tried to move a hand down to touch her cunt but the restraints prevented any movement. She cried out in frustration before feeling his fingers there, the pads of his fingertips tapping gently over her engorged and throbbing clit.

'Come for me, slut. Come with me buried in your arse. Come for your Master.'

Her orgasm had already taken hold, and she contracted violently around nothing, the emptiness in her cunt only emphasising the contractions in her arse. Feeling her spasm around his rock-hard cock was too much, and he began spilling his seed deep into her bowels. He grunted into her ear as he came, called her a dirty fucking bitch, telling her he loved her, that he owned her, that she belonged to him. Her own orgasm was still rife, and, with these words and the feeling of him spurting jets of hot come into her, she came again, tearfully sobbing as her body reached its limit.

Finally, after forever, they collapsed onto the bed, him still inside her and both their bodies racked with sweat, come and tears. He slithered out of her arse, and they soon fell fast asleep with his come dribbling slowly out of her. It was her favourite way to sleep.

J B, age 30
Homosexual
Single, moderately sexually active
No children
College degree
Occupation unknown
Arizona, USA

I would like to have six women at once (one on each hand, one on each foot, one on my mouth, one giving me head) while underwater. This is obviously a fantasy because of a human need for air.

Maggie, age 18
Heterosexual
Virgin
High School student
Ohio, USA

When I was young (er, I'm not old now), I was very closed-minded. *Everything* offended me, especially bondage, which was ironic considering my idol for both my confidence and my body was Bettie Page. When I discovered she was popular for her bondage work (naive, much?) I was a little disturbed, but I started to become more accepting. If Bettie did it, then it must not be as evil/weird as I'd been led to think. Then, a few years ago, I saw the movie *Secretary* and found myself distressingly turned on. So I started poking around the internet, reading related books (*Story of O, Venus in Furs*; I avoided, and still do, Sade, because I find him tasteless), and finding whatever movies I could on the subject. I went from missionary, vanilla, maybe a few strawberries thrown in for good measure, to chains, whips and leather in a matter of months. Now anything with a touch of domination to it is enough to get me a little hot. Maybe it's the alpha male in the vampire romance book, or maybe it's the possessive lover in the vanilla ones. Movies, too, that reference bondage or D/s, are huge turn-ons. And leather clothes, of course!

All the men I know are pussies. It doesn't help that I'm stuck in the middle of super-Christian Ohio, where the boys get this wide-eyed look and consider running home to mommy if you even hint at wanting to be tied up. That, and I'm very romantic – I'm still a virgin because I don't really want to even play until I'm in love. Maybe not first love; I don't want to jump right in the sack with the first guy I've got feelings for. I want to be a little sane about it, you know?

The themes of my fantasies involve bondage, being dominated, and S&M in general. This usually all occurs in an M/s sort of setting. And I can never fantasise if there isn't love involved, so it's usually a committed and very fictional relationship. I'm a feminist's dream, I'll tell you that. So usually my fantasies involve the same characters – I'm a writer, so I like consistency in my cast. My favourite usually involves a dom character of mine (Tiberius, also my favourite) sneaking up on me and blindfolding me, then asking me to strip. He leads me to his room and lays me gently face down on the four-poster bed; then he ties me up, spreadeagled, and gives me a massage.

Nice warm peppermint oil; candles that I can't see but I can smell; lovely low light, maybe some music.

Then out comes the knife.

Sometimes he'll excuse himself for a moment while he goes to get himself a glass of wine; other times he'll already have it somewhere on his person, or on the end table. He teases me – it might be sharp, it might not. I'm terrified of blades and cuts, so I do as he says and stay stiff as a board, terror and desire all welling up in a delicious combination as he drags the tip of the blade over my skin: my thighs, my back, the back of my neck, the backs of my arms. Sometimes he presses hard enough to draw welts over me. Then, when I'm least expecting it and soaked from the fear, he slides it between my thighs (his finger over the edge if it is, indeed, the sharp knife) and fucks me with it. When I first realise just what he's done, I whimper and try to squirm away, but he warns me that any undue movement and I'll hurt myself.

Oh, yeah, and he's laughing the whole time, sometimes leaning down to kiss me and tell me how proud he is or how much he loves me.

Damn, now I need to change my panties.

Sue, age 43
Bisexual
Live-in relationship/marriage
Children
College
Dream Interpreter
Southeast Scotland, UK

On discovering an S&M magazine at the age of eight, I discovered that it gave me a 'strange' feeling. As I grew up I realised that this feeling was sexual excitement! I am now in a D/s relationship with my partner, with me being the submissive one. I'm more at ease with who and what I am, and have become an active member of the BDSM community.

In my fantasy I am lying naked on the bitter stone; I can feel the carvings beneath me pressing themselves into my flesh. As I turn my head I can see those same symbols cut into the monoliths that surround this slab I'm chained to.

I move my head again, staring up at the moon, full and glistening in the clear night sky. A slight breeze whispers over my nudity and my nipples stiffen. In the distance I can hear a single drumbeat repeating over and over and over, the seconds counting down until my fate is realised.

I hear him approach, his footfalls muffled by the damp grass. I dare not turn to look at him and instead close my eyes and view his features from the scorching on my memory.

I feel his aura spiral with mine as he moves his hand just above my body. I yearn for him to touch me, to feel the warmth of his hand just one more time. He senses my thoughts and places his hand, fingers spread, on my chest, the heel of his hand taking in my increasing heartbeat.

In a swift movement, his hand grips my throat, his forefinger and thumb squeezing into my neck. Leaning down, I feel his sweet breath on my face, know that my lips are parting slightly in anticipation of his kiss. And when that comes I sigh so deeply, immersing myself in him.

I feel bereaved as he pulls away from the kiss. His fingers move from my throat and trail lightly down the length of my body, his fingers exploring my slit, gathering my moisture then anointing my lips with those juices.

He tells me to open my eyes, to let him see my love, my commitment, my devotion. I gaze up at him and feel myself drowning in his exquisiteness.

I catch a reflection in his eyes, the glint of metal, then feel a needlepoint of steel press lightly at the side of my neck. I know the time has come. The end and the beginning. There is no pain as he draws the knife over my throat, only a deep sense of joy, an ever-increasing warmth inside me. I feel my eyelids flutter and I begin the eternal journey that he has sent me on.

Rough Trade

Lucia, age 36
Heterosexual
Live-in relationship/marriage
No children
Bachelor's degree
Homemaker
Northeast England, UK

I'm turned on by any form of punishment, especially spanking, the display of legitimate authority of one person over another. To be honest, actual sex is never all that arousing to me. I live completely in my head, so my fantasies are the mind-blowing part for me, not the physical sensations of sex. I don't find anything offensive when it comes to an individual's personal fantasies. There are no taboos in the safety and freedom of fantasy; nor should there be.

This is my most embarrassing confession and I've never shared it with anyone. I have a recurring fantasy about being selected for special experiments in a Nazi prison camp. I'm sent to a 'love camp' to be a whore for the officers of the Third Reich. Some men have more sadistic desires than others, and girls who fail to satisfy are punished. After a public whipping in the yard, they are left naked in bondage afterwards, on display as an example to the others. One of my favourite embellishments is an officer who stops to look at the marks after I've been whipped. He says, 'Looks like someone's been a naughty girl', and fondles me casually while I moan in shame.

One day a scientist arrives and all the girls are lined up in the yard for inspection. He needs a girl for a special experiment. He makes his way down the line, opening the girls' tops and fondling their breasts, lifting their skirts and touching them, commenting to his assistant who follows with a clipboard. It's all very businesslike, like a slave auction. I whimper and squirm at his touch when it's my turn, and he likes my responsiveness. 'I'll take this one,' he says at last. 'Have her cleaned up and brought to my laboratory.'

After a thorough, invasive and humiliating medical examination, I am used as a guinea pig for different methods of punishment. He doesn't talk to me at all – only to his assistant. First he straps me down on my back on a sterile tilting table. My arms are secured overhead. He unbuttons my top to expose my breasts for a whipping. Next I am strapped down over a trestle and he uses a cane on my bottom. Sometimes he leaves the room and his assistant molests me – he's not as duty-minded as his superior.

Tracy, age 49
Heterosexual
Steady relationship, not live-in
Children
BSN
Nurse
Birmingham, UK

I generally have BDSM fantasies. I am submissive and they usually involve both male and female doms. I have in the past fantasised about gang-bangs and other women. In my favourite fantasy I'm naked in a corner with my hands on my head. My female dom ushers in three men. They ignore me, spending time looking at photos of previous sessions and discussing what will happen during this session, which will culminate in me being anally fucked by all three men. I am summoned by the mistress to the centre of the room and slowly spanked, paddled, and caned until I'm highly marked ... nipple clamps, etc., are used. After a break where my marks are admired by all present, my mistress uses a large dildo to mouth-fuck me and spreads my legs to show the men that I'm in fact enjoying it very much. She inserts the dildo in my cunt and directs the men to fuck my ass very hard. I say thank you.

Name withheld, age 25
Heterosexual
Live-in relationship/marriage
Children
A level
Logistics Administrator
Cheshire, England

I usually fantasise once a day. I'm now a lot more open to different sexual preferences and will try anything once; I keep an open mind. What holds me back is the fear of shocking my husband! My current favourite fantasy is about being urinated on during sex – to be made to drink my tormentor's pee, to have him pee in every hole, and the entire time he's telling me how bad and naughty I am.

Louise, age 45
Heterosexual
Live-in relationship/marriage
College degree
Journalist
Northwest England, UK

From the earliest times (aged ten or eleven) I was drawn to bondage and submission. I have no idea where it came from. My background was pretty normal/average and these fantasies arrived out of the blue. At seventeen, I came across *The Story of O*, which encapsulated my fantasies completely and has remained the basis for everything since then. I fought my desires for a long time and I was 28 before I finally plucked up the courage to accept my sexuality.

My fantasies revolve entirely around BDSM and being used as a sex slave. My lover takes me to a country house one night. On arrival, we are met by the lady of the house and I discover it is a high-class swingers club. I am taken to an anteroom where I'm ordered to strip except for my stockings and heels. My lover laces a skin-tight leather hood on my head, and adds leather wrist and ankle cuffs. I am nervous but excited. He leads me out of the anteroom, down corridors – I can hear voices all around me, some commenting on me and wondering who the woman in the hood is. We arrive in another room. He tells me to sit on the bed. I can tell it is large and has satin sheets. He stands very close to me and speaks into my ear loudly (so I can hear through the leather) – he is going to sell me that night to anyone who wants to fuck me. I will not see any of my 'customers'. I sit nervously, heart pounding. Almost immediately, I hear the door open and people coming in. Someone pinches my nipples hard and tells me I have nice tits. I can't hear much though. There are hands touching my body.

I am pushed back on the bed and a man climbs on top of me. His hard cock goes straight in, I am so wet. Someone turns my head and forces his large, hard cock into my mouth through the mouth hole of the hood. I start to suck him. He shoots into my mouth at the same time as the other man spunks into my cunt. Almost immediately, I am turned over and made to kneel. The cuffs on my wrists and ankles are fastened to the bed and now I'm completely trapped. I feel lube being smeared into my arsehole and then I am violated there too. Once again my mouth is not spared.

The evening continues in this way – one man after another, sometimes several at the same time, each using me as they want. My lover allows me little breaks occasionally, during which he twists my nipples and spanks me hard or canes me and lets me know how pleased he is with me. I am grateful for his touch and knowing that he's there watching over me. Then the fucking and sucking resumes. I lose track of time. It's pitch-dark inside the hood and hot – the hood is so tight, and I revel in its anonymity. At one point I am made to sit astride a huge cock while another man enters my arse and yet another my mouth. Even my hands are not spared as two more thrusting erections insist on being wanked. Every hole is used relentlessly, with barely any time in between to recover from each violation. I am tiring and sweating but there is no let-up. How many men have had me? I cannot tell anymore. On the next break, I plead with my lover for mercy but am rewarded only with another hard caning that just makes me even wetter. My cunt juices and the wads of anonymous spunk dribble out of my cunt and arse and run down my legs. My stockings are damp and sticky. I have swallowed at least twenty mouthfuls of come.

Finally, I feel my lover's hands on me, gently caressing me and telling me I have been a good girl. Now it is his turn. He removes the cuffs from my wrists and ankles but leaves the hood on. I feel soft cotton rope on my body as he expertly ties me into Japanese bondage that forces my tender tits into a tight thrust-upwards position. My ankles are tied to my thighs, leaving me wide open, and I am helpless. He inserts a dildo gag into my mouth and now I am silenced too. He slaps my breasts hard, twists the nipples yet again, then puts clover clamps on them. He inserts his fingers into my cunt. I am so wet and open, he can get three in easily. Then he works in another finger. He pushes his fingers in and out, fucking me with his hand. Then I feel his thumb start to slide in too. Slowly, slowly, he works his entire hand into me until I am impaled on his fist. I am longing to come as that has been denied me all night. And now I'm focused entirely on his fist in my cunt and its slow but unrelenting movement inside me. Despite all the cocks I have taken, this is the first time tonight I have felt truly filled up and this is the only one that matters as it is him. He works his hand until I am desperate for release. I try to tell him I want to come but I'm muffled by the gag. Suddenly, I feel a buzzing sensation on my aching clit – a vibrator. It takes very little to tip me over the edge and I spasm violently around his fist as I scream into the gag. My orgasm ends and another one starts as he holds the vibrator hard against me. I come again, then starts a third, then a fourth orgasm. On the fifth one, I piss myself as I come hard for the last time. I lie back exhausted in my own wetness as my lover gently slips his fist out of my shattered cunt. He unties me and holds me tight, telling me he loves me. Then he leads me out of the bedroom, still wearing the hood, and back to the anteroom. There he dresses me, and leads me out of the club. Only when we are back in the car does he finally remove the hood. As we drive off, he tells me I was used by more than sixty men and that I earned a lot of money – he gives me the wad of cash and tells me that next time he is going to give me away rather than pimp me.

Name withheld, age 24
Heterosexual
Live-in relationship/marriage
No children
Student/Part-time Retail
Missouri, USA

I don't even know how long I've been masturbating, fantasising, and having orgasms, but it's been at least since I was five. When I was fairly young (probably eight or nine), I'd think about getting spanked while I rubbed myself against a pillow. I'd think a lot about touching other girls and women. I didn't think about intercourse, because the concept seemed so foreign. All I knew of sex was masturbation and nudity. And just a little bit of pain. Every time I saw coercion or BDSM on TV or in movies, I'd always be turned on by the imagery. We might not think about it anymore, but, when I was a kid, I managed to see lots of instances of rough and kinky sex. There are allusions to it on TV, certainly, and it pops up in movies. I wasn't a sheltered kid, so I got to see a lot of really great movies with some very adult themes. I'd get angry at myself, but rape scenes in movies often turned me on.

Titanic came out just as my sexuality was blooming, and that movie really moistened my young teen panties. The idea that anyone could find me beautiful, so beautiful that I had to be drawn nude, was irresistible. I grew up as the fat kid, and never imagined that anyone would find my body attractive or desirable. The idea of sex so saturated with romance was very appealing. Oh, you're shaking as you fuck me in this buggy-like car? I'll hold you. I'll soothe you, I would fantasise.

Every time I see a woman having an orgasm in mainstream media (which, by the way, doesn't happen nearly enough), I am so turned on. Meg Ryan has a fake orgasm in *When Harry Met Sally*, and I get wet. Porn where the focus is female pleasure turns me on, but this can be hard to find. That's why I really enjoy squirters because, well, she's probably not faking. Men going down on women, either in mainstream media or porn, really turns me on. I more fully enjoy porn when I know that the woman is having a good time.

It seems like, aside from those teen hormone fantasies involving Johnny Depp or Leonardo DiCaprio sweeping me away and fucking me on a private beach, I've always seemed to have kinky fantasies, especially spanking. Pornography and erotica have definitely pushed the boundary of my fantasy world. In my teens I might have imagined close-ups of genitals while fucking. When I first began seeing porn in college, it was as if the fantasy were fulfilled. I knew what it looked like. Of course, I still fantasise about a lot of things that you can regularly see in porn, like anal. Erotica, especially, has opened up my fantasy world to unusual and kinky things – things I would never fantasise about acting on or being involved with, but what I still find hot is slavery, heavy BDSM, incest, mind control, group sex and bukkake.

I'm so turned on when my husband cleans the house, fixes the car, or runs errands. I just want to drop to my knees and suck his balls dry, which gets me very wet. I'm turned on when I get touched on certain areas of my body, when my husband tells me I'm beautiful, and listens to what I have to say. I'm turned on when our friends talk about their sex lives. It's almost like a sex urge for competition's sake. I'm turned on by porn that's either about female pleasure or degradation, like when a man is forceful and dominant, either in or out of a BDSM setting ... but, you know, in a sexy way.

Often I fantasise in 'themes'. I have dominance themes, where I imagine someone, usually my husband, controlling me. Sometimes it's spanking, sometimes it's humiliation, sometimes it's bondage. I have a dirty motel room fantasy theme where anything goes, but often with women involved. I have a romance theme where I imagine those emotionally satisfying sexual moments in my life where I felt closeness and love, where the sex is tender and intimate. I have rape fantasies where men tie me up, use a knife to cut off my clothes, fuck me hard (until I come, natch), then come on my face, hair or tits.

I'm married and we're monogamous and, unfortunately, I'm the kinky one in the relationship. My husband will indulge some of my fantasies, but we don't do it very often, usually on special occasions. I'm not saying I mind. I wouldn't want kinky sex all the time, just once or twice a month, something to fantasise about later. This is rather common for me, fantasising about the things I've done already. We've gone so far as to do light bondage, a little bit of spanking, a little bit of name-calling. I don't know that I've ever told him that my fantasies run deeper than that, but I've always assumed he knows that they are more intense. It's an unspoken rule that he acknowledges my kinks and will occasionally indulge me, but isn't interested himself, other than for my own pleasure. We've discussed BDSM issues, and I've explained concepts to him before. We've discussed, in a broad sense, restraints, gags, safe words, nipple clamps, and many other things that we haven't done. I'd like very much to act on these fantasies, but realise I'll probably get the same reaction: 'Well, maybe for your birthday', or 'I don't want to do that, so how about I just tie you up?' That's why I don't discuss them in detail, because of the rejection I might face.

It's not as if my sex life is otherwise unfulfilling, I'd just like to have a little more kink.

In my favourite fantasy there's a man at my house, and he's angry. I've done something rather distasteful, the details of what aren't important, and he wants to punish me. He will, however, reserve the bulk of his cruelty for when we are both naked. If we were clothed, my feminist sensibilities wouldn't put up with his bullshit. When I'm naked, though, his anger is arousing.

He asks me to undress, though he, of course, stays clothed. He leers at my naked body, eyeing me like a piece of meat. I'm supposed to bend over his lap, which I do, and he gives my ass many hard swats. It stings and, each time he slaps, I hear a hard treble 'clap'. He waits just long enough for the sting to subside a little, then swats my ass just a little harder. He's spanking me and, while he does it, reminds me how badly I've misbehaved, and reminds me of what a slut I am. No fantasy would be complete without the demeaning names: bitch, slut, whore.

He makes me crawl around on my hands and knees while he makes quick work of shedding his clothes. I crawl in front of him; he grabs me by the back of the head and fucks my throat. In fantasyland, my deep throat is impeccable. Next he ties me up and fucks me. Sometimes he's tied my hands, fucking me doggy while slapping my ass. Sometimes he gags me, blindfolds me and fucks me missionary, whispering terrible things in my ear. Sometimes he 'makes' me get on top, orders me not to make a noise, and frequently tells me to hop off and suck his cock.

Eventually he'll come on my face, reminding me that sluts don't get to come (man, that *really* gets me off), then makes me lick up any last drops of come off the floor. Get the floor really clean, he reminds me, his huge hand resting on my neck.

If I haven't come yet by this point in the fantasy, he might make me go out without wiping the come off my face, or he might tie me up and cause me a little pain. He might get so hot by looking at my face glazed with come that he gets hard again, fucks my face (reminding me, again, that sluts don't get to come) and comes directly in my throat.

Amy, age 26
Bisexual
Single, very sexually active
A levels
Student
Yorkshire, UK

I imagine being young, fourteen or fifteen, and being a true Lolita-type girl. I imagine seducing countless men and allowing them to abuse, humiliate and rape me. Submission to a man turns me on, being controlled, abused, humiliated, hurt ... but then being treated respectfully and with tenderness afterwards! Personal fantasies are a huge turn-on. I've begun to know myself more and more in the past year. Until that point, I was frustrated and bored with sex – it seemed to promise much, but deliver very little. Average sex is not for me – I know that. I have also discovered that there's no shame in succumbing to your most secret desires; repression is something the English are too good at, and it's bad for the soul and the development, I believe. I held myself back and caused damage to myself because culture and society were at work on my brain, telling me that I was a deviant and a freak! – when all along I was just a bit ... alternative and experimental! To be honest, the most rewarding and fulfilling sexual experiences, for me, have not involved out-and-out sex. They have been more exercises in control and manipulation.

Living out my fantasy would interfere with my daily life! My ultimate fantasy is to be a slave to a Master in a full-time power-exchange relationship ... but I also want/need to study, write, think, read, be, etc.! This is a piece I wrote, then showed to my boyfriend. We then acted it out for real. That was pretty good and we stuck accurately to the fantasy. What a treat!

You are driving and I am sitting beside you. According to your specification, I have worn fishnet tights, a tiny black dress and make-up. It is night and it's raining. There is very little visible outside bar smudges of fluorescent light, bleary-eyed headlamps and water. We have the distinct impression it has always been raining and night. I am warm, and enjoying you sitting next to me. You make a wonderful driver, and I feel privileged to be in a position to appreciate you drive. Perhaps this sounds ridiculous, but it's true. You are a calm driver, knowing where everything is about you; you are in full control of your every movement and action. You are considered, and I love to consider your manners and ways. You are on display, showing off to me, and yet you don't fully realise the effect you are having. The sight of your hands on the steering wheel makes me hot. Your movements, the outline of your fingers, your carefully cut cuticles, your tense grip followed by a fluid gear change makes me even hotter. Every time you breathe you turn me on, the sight of your lips alone makes me wet between the legs. I have brought scissors, tape, rope, a hair-brush, a collar and a lead.

I cannot help staring at your hands: their size, weight and texture fascinate me. Never before have I truly considered a man to be beautiful, but you are. Never before have I unquestioningly believed every word that one person uttered so unconditionally. Your legs are beautifully long, and black trousers accentuate your powerful aura. You were made to wear smart suits and jackets and well-cut trousers. Your torso is awesome, long and awesome, your powerful neck, your jaw line, your stubble ... the sight of your body makes me hot and wet all over. Fluid seeps out into the crotch of my fishnets and makes them sticky and damp against my legs and cunt. I cannot take my eyes off your hands; I dream about taking them inside me, and having them prod, probe, finger, screw, smear, jab, slap, punch, poke, twist, grab and fuck around with my body. I want your fingers to know my body from every possible angle, avenue and orifice; to push and pull it around, abuse, ravage, wreck, disfigure, distort and mangle it. I want you to wreak havoc on my body, use it as you want: to play with, dismantle, poke into and pull apart. I want you inside me in every possible way, and then I want you to break out and leave me somewhere, or nowhere, to start from again.

The rain continues pelting the windscreen at the same pace. We come to a standstill and the fluorescent lights stop moving; they are static blobs, like fucked-up versions of paintings by Pollock, or Miró, who I had always assumed was a woman. I long to touch your cock. I want to stroke your trousers, place my hand on your hardness, feel the strength of your desire to hurt me and fuck me. I want to make it harder. I stare straight ahead and focus on the night before us; this is my first opportunity to please you fully and give you the true level of submission that you deserve.

Eventually we join a ring road and drive into the city centre. It is strangely quiet, but then pockets of life emerge at intervals and we pass by them with a sense of estrangement. You drive directly to the hotel, and we pull up in the underground car park. Your hands are placed flat on your thighs, and I have absolutely no idea what you are thinking, except a vague notion that your thoughts will involve fairly intense levels of violation and transgression. The knowledge of this makes me instantly wet and we leave the car, collecting our bags from the boot.

The foyer is ultra modern and full of curves – curved booths and sofas, marble pillars, and nondescript sculptures on curved plinths. Cameras follow each person who walks through the revolving doors, and a few businessmen lurk on the curved sofas, trying to exude danger and money. The reception is decked out in swathes of plush material, and ambient lighting is the order of the day. Irrelevant and insipid Muzak plays everywhere, being transmitted through a myriad of hidden speakers. A rather incongruous rock pool is stage left of the reception desk, replete with ferns, waterfalls and lizards on the rocks.

A bellboy sidles up to us and collects our bags as we check in. We follow him up to our room in one of those extremely modern lifts that makes no sound whatsoever.

'If you require or desire anything, absolutely anything, I am at your service,' says the bellboy.

He shows us to our room: 419.

The youth leaves and we dump down our bags.

'Stay there,' you say, and then you walk over to the blood-red curtains and look out of the window. The city stands below.

'Are you ready, cunt?'

'Yes, Master.'

'Are you ready to demonstrate your submission to me? To obey me without question or hesitation? To comply as readily as you can, and truly succumb to my will, to make my will your own will, and to experience my desire as your own desire?'

'I am ready, Master.'

You go to the bag in the corner of the room and take out a thick leather collar with rings around it. You walk towards me, holding the collar flat on your open palms.

'Lift up your hair, whore.'

You bring the collar up to my neck and wrap it around me, moving behind me as you do so. The feel of the heavy leather pressing against my skin and then being fitted tightly around my neck makes my cunt throb. My cunt feels like an entity outside of myself. You fasten the collar and place your hands on my shoulders. Your presence behind me is thrilling; your cock is inches away from my ass. You remove your hands and then go once more to the bag. This time you take out a leather lead, and again walk towards me, holding it over your outspread palms. Your hands turn me on unbelievably.

'Kiss your lead, cunt.'

I kiss my lead, and you attach it to one of the rings on the collar. You step back and look pleased. I smile at you, and you smile back, holding the end of the lead.

'On your hands and knees, pig.'

I get down on hands and knees, my dress moving up my body and showing off my ass. You pull on the lead and walk towards the bathroom. I follow, dutifully, on my hands and knees, my cunt pulsing for you with your every step. I can see your calves through your trousers, and delight in their movement beneath the material. Your body fascinates me. Your bones, your skin, your manners and movements hold an endless pull. You have drawn me like a map, or a constellation. I am a new land which pleases you and exists to serve you.

You take me into the bathroom. It is stark and bright and tiled. A night on the tiles appeals to me. You lift up the toilet lid.

'Lick the rim, cunt.'

I lean over the bowl and begin rapidly licking the circumference of the bowl's rim. It is not shit or piss that makes me retch but cleaning products. Shit or piss would be preferable. I gag on the taste and smell of the chemicals but continue licking around the rim. You watch me gag and it pleases you.

'Keep licking, cunt.'

I carry on, filled with satisfaction that you are enjoying yourself. I lick around either side of the rim and nearly puke, retching into the toilet bowl. You slip the lead's loop around your wrist, unzip your trousers and take out your cock. You grab a fistful of hair and pull on it, tightening your grip on it. You yank my head back and then pull it over the toilet bowl, flipping me over onto my back. You arch my back over the side of the bowl and then hold your cock over my face and piss all over my hair and face, then shoot it right into my mouth. I swallow every drop gladly, watching your face as you empty yourself into me. You let go of my hair and move your fingers around my neck and squeeze. Your hand almost completely encircles my neck and it makes me hot and wet across my body. You shake me with your hand and throttle me as the last shakes of your piss slide down my tightened throat. Your grip is fierce and the tighter you hold me the wetter I get. My cunt is aching for you. Again, you flip me over so that my face is inside the toilet bowl. You shove my head down into the bottom of the bowl.

'Lap up that toilet water, you fucking bitch.'

I drink up the water and you flush the toilet and hold down my head, gripping onto the sides of my neck with your fingers, pinching into me so that I gag all over again. The water bubbles up, completely swamping my face. I am immersed in the water and about to puke. The bubbling subsides and you lift up my head and look at my face, delighting in the streams of mascara and splotches of smudged lipstick across my cheeks. Your satisfaction fills me with desire. Again you push my face into the water and flush the toilet. The bubbles billow up inside my mouth and I can barely breathe. The water floods into my throat and down into my body. As the flushing subsides I retch and puke into the bowl. You hold my hair back and shake my head as the vomit falls out of my body.

When you have shaken the vomit from my body, you lift me up and I sit up straight on my knees.

'Now, bitch, lick up the piss from the floor.'

I bend down and lap up the spilled piss from the tiles. You push onto the back of my head with your foot, shoving my face against the floor and I lap harder at the pools of liquid, drinking up your piss till the floor is completely clean.

'Now what do you say, cunt?'

'Thank you, Master.'

'Good. On your hands and knees.'

I resume my position on the floor, my hair dripping with piss and dregs of puke. You lead me back into the bedroom.

'Sit cross-legged on the floor at the foot of the bed.'

I do as I am told and sit like a good girl with my hands on my lap. You walk over to the phone on the table by the side of the bed and order a bottle of champagne from room service. I feel filthy and adore the feeling. I want you to make me feel filthy, make me do disgusting things. I want to do disgusting things: you allow me to do them. You are my Master, in charge of my own descent into filth, choosing the disgusting acts I must perform. I will always perform them to the best of my ability. I want you to show me how disgusting I can be, push me into the rectum of filth, dream up sick and nasty tasks for me, give me dreams of filth and service; I will do it all, you will drive and direct me. I want to know my own pleasure and yours and construct them in parallel, assemble them together.

You stand in front of me.

'Pick up your lead and give it to me, pig.'

I hand you the end of the lead and look up at you.

'Up onto your knees, cunt, and hands behind your head.'

I do it and you slap me around the face five times, quickly and hard.

'Lift up your dress.'

I do as I am told and you punch me in the stomach twice. The combination of surprise and pain makes me even hotter.

'Are you wet?' you ask.

'Incredibly,' I reply.

A knock comes at the door, which prompts you to remove my lead and collar.

'Stand up and hands by your side.'

I comply. You take the hairbrush out of the bag and comb through my hair, pushing it back out of my face. You lick your thumb and wipe away the smears of make-up and then stand back.

'Now you're going to prove what a slut you really are.'

The knock comes again.

'You're going to let this bellboy fuck you, cunt, and I'm going to watch from behind the bathroom door. Don't let him see me, pig.'

You walk into the bathroom and pull the door closed, leaving enough of a gap so that I can see you and you can see the bed. I walk towards the sound of the knocking, open the door and smile sweetly.

'Hello, come in.'

Samantha, age 36
Bisexual
Live-in relationship/marriage and steady relationships, not live-in
Education and occupation unknown
London, UK

Anyone who treated me badly or told me what to do turned me on. Someone once held a knife to my throat in bed and, although he wasn't playing at all (he'd heard a rumour about me and wanted to know if it was true), it was possibly the most exciting experience I'd ever had at the time. I must have been fourteen or fifteen at the most (I'm afraid I started pretty early!). I'm still turned on by anyone who can dominate me or who seems like they might be able to (Vic Mackey from

The Shield, for example … oooh, yes please! Not exactly gorgeous but sooo masterful!). As for things, it's all the same theme really. Any kind of control equipment, restraints, cuffs, collars (especially collars), even just a length of rope and anything that'll probably hurt some while I'm restrained – floggers, paddles, clamps, even a humble clothes peg. When it comes to particular experiences, I'm mad for having my hair pulled or my face slapped or just being forced to do something, anything really. I always say that it would turn me on to paint the bathroom ceiling on one leg if someone told me to do it in the right tone of voice, although I've never actually put this theory to the test! It's the words that really do it for me; I love the talking, I get much more turned on by someone telling me what they're going to do to me than if they just got on and did it! I sometimes think it would be easier if I was turned on by romance and a massage but I'm not so there's no point wishing, is there? I just have to accept that I am what I am and make the best of it. But it can make life difficult sometimes.

My fantasies involve the themes of domination, submission (mine), pain, control, and lately water sports too, but tied in with the BDSM theme. There's usually lots of, 'No, no, please, Master, don't make me do it, please no, no!' Doesn't matter what it's about, just the begging will get me going.

In my fantasy my Master has decided that today he's going to take me further than ever before. He says he's bought me a present and that I'm to kneel in front of him on the floor to receive it. He tells me to put my hands out flat in front of me and then places a cane in my palms.

I cry out as I know what will be coming next and I tell him that I'm not ready for this yet, I'm only just getting used to our flogger and to step up to a cane is too much, too soon.

He tells me that he knows it's what I've always wanted, to

see welts on my body and he's sick of hearing me complain that I want more from him. He's warned me before to be careful what I wish for and now he's going to give me what I claim to want.

'Now we'll see,' he says.

'Yes, Master,' I am forced to reply, knowing that what he says is true but still being terrified of the instrument.

He says that I have to ask him to use it on me but I can't get the words out. I cry and beg him not to do this but he remains unmoved, eventually silencing me with the words 'Hush now.'

I manage to ask him to use the cane and he bids me to present it to him on my open palms. He takes it from me but has me leave my hands where they are.

'Close your eyes and keep them closed,' he says seriously, and I realise what's coming. He pauses before striking my hands with the cane and I cry out in pain.

'Be quiet!' he commands and continues to hit my palms at random intervals so that I cannot anticipate the next blow. After a while he tells me he's done and through my sobs I thank him for my pain.

Just when I think it's over he pulls me to my feet by my hair and fastens my wrists to the chains in our bedroom ceiling. I know what he's going to do and become all but hysterical, crying and begging him not to put me through this.

He ignores my pleas and goes about the job of getting me ready, locking the cuffs and forcing my feet apart with the spreader bar.

Then, without warning, he strikes my arse and I scream. He strokes the hair back from my face and tells me not to make a sound again unless he tells me I can.

I bite my lip to try to keep quiet as he beats me, sometimes softly with quick little taps, then sometimes hard in heavy single blows on my arse or my tits or my (by-now dripping wet) pussy.

After a while he holds my head up with my hair so that I look at him and strokes my cheek gently. He says that he is going to ask me if I've had enough but that I am to say 'no'. He says that when he asks if I want him to stop I am to say 'no' and that when he checks that I want more I am to say 'yes'.

I am still crying and pleading with him not to and eventually I ask him why he is doing this to me. He says calmly, as if explaining to a child, that I know why, it's because I *need* it. I need to suffer for him, to make me whole.

This calms me down a little as deep down I know he is right, so when he asks if I've had enough yet, I am able to say a little shakily, 'No, Master, thank you', and, when he asks if he should stop now, I repeat a bit more confidently, 'No, Master, thank you', and then, when he finally says, 'Do you want more then?', I clearly say, 'Yes please, Master'.

'Yes please, Master, what?'

'Please Master, please hurt me with the cane some more.'

'Why?'

I pause before slowly admitting it. 'Because I need you to, Master.'

So he strikes me again and again and again, leaving vicious-looking stripes all over my body, and I cry, not so much from the pain now but from the knowledge of what I have just admitted.

Eventually he releases me and I collapse into his arms still sobbing, I say sorry over and over again, for not doing well, but he tells me what a good girl I am and how proud he is of me and smothers me with little kisses, holding me tight and stroking my hair until I am calm.

LOOK OUT FOR THE BLACK LACE 15TH ANNIVERSARY SPECIAL EDITIONS. COLLECT ALL 10 TITLES IN THE SERIES!

All books priced £7.99 in the UK. Please note publication dates apply to the UK only. For other territories, please contact your retailer.

Published in March 2008

CASSANDRA'S CONFLICT
Fredrica Allen
ISBN 978 0 352 34186 0

A house in Hampstead. Present day. Behind a façade of cultured respectability lies a world of decadent indulgence and dark eroticism. Cassandra's sheltered life is transformed when she gets employed as governess to the Baron's children. He draws her into games where lust can feed on the erotic charge of submission. Games where only he knows the rules and where unusual pleasures can flourish.

To be published in April 2008

GEMINI HEAT
Portia Da Costa
ISBN 978 0 352 34187 7

As the metropolis sizzles in the freak early summer temperatures, identical twin sisters Deana and Delia Ferraro are cooking up a heat wave of their own. Surrounded by an atmosphere of relentless humidity, Deanna and Delia find themselves rivals for the attentions of Jackson de Guile – an exotic, wealthy entrepreneur and master of power dynamics – who draws them both into a web of luxurious debauchery.

Their erotic encounters become increasingly bizarre as the twins vie for the rewards that pleasuring him brings them – tainted rewards which only serve to confuse their perceptions of the limits of sexual experience.

To be published in May 2008

BLACK ORCHID
Roxanne Carr
ISBN 978 0 352 34188 4

At the Black Orchid Club, adventurous women who yearn for the pleasures of exotic, even kinky, sex can quench their desires in discreet and luxurious surroundings. Having tasted the fulfilment of unique and powerful lusts, one such adventurous woman learns what happens when the need for limitless indulgence becomes an addiction.

To be published in June 2008

FORBIDDEN FRUIT
Susie Raymond
ISBN 978 0 352 34189 1

The last thing sexy thirty-something Beth expected was to get involved with a sixteen year old. But when she finds him spying on her in the dressing room at work she embarks on an erotic journey with the straining youth, teaching him and teasing him as she leads him through myriad sensuous exercises at her stylish modern home. As their lascivious games become more and more intense, Beth soon begins to realise that she is the one being awakened to a new world of desire – and that hers is the mind quickly becoming consumed with lust.

To be published in July 2008

JULIET RISING
Cleo Cordell
ISBN 978 0 352 34192 1

Nothing is more important to Reynard than winning the favours of the bright and wilful Juliet, a pupil at Madame Nicol's exclusive but strict 18th century ladies' academy. Her captivating beauty tinged with a hint of cruelty soon has Reynard willing to do anything to win her approval. But Juliet's methods have little effect on Andreas, the real object of her lustful obsessions. Unable to bend him to her will, she is forced to watch him lavish his manly talents on her fellow pupils. That is, until she agrees to change her stuck-up, stubborn ways and become an eager erotic participant.

To be published in August 2008

ODALISQUE
Fleur Reynolds
ISBN 978 0 352 34193 8

Set against a backdrop of sophisticated elegance, a tale of family intrigue, forbidden passions and depraved secrets unfolds. Beautiful but scheming, successful designer Auralie plots to bring about the downfall of her virtuous cousin, Jeanine. Recently widowed, but still young and glamorous, Jeanine finds her passions being rekindled by Auralie's husband. But she is playing into Auralie's hands – vindictive hands that drag Jeanine into a world of erotic depravity. Why are the cousins locked into this sexual feud? And what is the purpose of Jeanine's mysterious Confessor, and his sordid underground sect?

To be published in September 2008

THE STALLION
Georgina Brown
ISBN 978 0 352 34199 0

The world of showjumping is as steamy as it is competitive. Ambitious young rider Penny Bennett enters into a wager with her oldest rival and friend, Ariadne, to win her thoroughbred stallion, guaranteed to bring Penny money and success. But first she must attain the sponsorship and very personal attention of showjumping's biggest impresario, Alister Beaumont.

Beaumont's riding school, however, is not all it seems. There's the weird relationship between Alister and his cigar-smoking sister. And the bizarre clothes they want Penny to wear. But in this atmosphere of unbridled kinkiness, Penny is determined not only to win the wager but to discover the truth about Beaumont's strange hobbies.

To be published in October 2008

THE DEVIL AND THE DEEP BLUE SEA
Cheryl Mildenhall
ISBN 978 0 352 34200 3

When Hillary and her girlfriends rent a country house for their summer vacation, it is a pleasant surprise to find that its secretive and kinky owner – Darius Harwood – seems to be the most desirable man in the locale. That is, before Hillary meets Haldane, the blonde and beautifully proportioned Norwegian sailor who works nearby. Intrigued by the sexual allure of two very different men, Hillary can't resist exploring the possibilities on offer. But these opportunities for misbehaviour quickly lead her into a tricky situation for which a diffcult decision has to be made.

To be published in November 2008

THE NINETY DAYS OF GENEVIEVE
Lucinda Carrington
ISBN 978 0 352 34201 0

A ninety-day sex contract wasn't exactly what Genevieve Loften had in mind when she began business negotiations with the arrogant and attractive James Sinclair. As a career move she wanted to go along with it; the pay-off was potentially huge.

However, she didn't imagine that he would make her the star performer in a series of increasingly kinky and exotic fantasies. Thrown into a world of sexual misadventure, Genevieve learns how to balance her high-pressure career with the twilight world of fetishism and debauchery.

To be published in December 2008

THE GIFT OF SHAME
Sarah Hope-Walker
ISBN 978 0 352 34202 7

Sad, sultry Helen flies between London, Paris and the Caribbean chasing whatever physical pleasures she can get to tear her mind from a deep, deep loss. Her glamorous lifestyle and charged sensual escapades belie a widow's grief. When she meets handsome, rich Jeffrey she is shocked and yet intrigued by his masterful, domineering behaviour. Soon, Helen is forced to confront the forbidden desires hiding within herself – and forced to undergo a startling metamorphosis from a meek and modest lady into a bristling, voracious wanton.

Black Lace Booklist

Information is correct at time of printing. To avoid disappointment, check availability before ordering. Go to www.black-lace-books.com.
All books are priced £7.99 unless another price is given.

BLACK LACE BOOKS WITH A CONTEMPORARY SETTING

☐ THE ANGELS' SHARE Maya Hess	ISBN 978 0 352 34043 6	
☐ ASKING FOR TROUBLE Kristina Lloyd	ISBN 978 0 352 33362 9	
☐ BLACK LIPSTICK KISSES Monica Belle	ISBN 978 0 352 33885 3	£6.99
☐ THE BLUE GUIDE Carrie Williams	ISBN 978 0 352 34132 7	
☐ CAMPAIGN HEAT Gabrielle Marcola	ISBN 978 0 352 33941 6	
☐ CAT SCRATCH FEVER Sophie Mouette	ISBN 978 0 352 34021 4	
☐ CIRCUS EXCITE Nikki Magennis	ISBN 978 0 352 34033 7	
☐ CLUB CRÈME Primula Bond	ISBN 978 0 352 33907 2	£6.99
☐ CONFESSIONAL Judith Roycroft	ISBN 978 0 352 33421 3	
☐ CONTINUUM Portia Da Costa	ISBN 978 0 352 33120 5	
☐ DANGEROUS CONSEQUENCES Pamela Rochford	ISBN 978 0 352 33185 4	
☐ DARK DESIGNS Madelynne Ellis	ISBN 978 0 352 34075 7	
☐ THE DEVIL INSIDE Portia Da Costa	ISBN 978 0 352 32993 6	
☐ EQUAL OPPORTUNITIES Mathilde Madden	ISBN 978 0 352 34070 2	
☐ FIRE AND ICE Laura Hamilton	ISBN 978 0 352 33486 2	
☐ GONE WILD Maria Eppie	ISBN 978 0 352 33670 5	
☐ HOTBED Portia Da Costa	ISBN 978 0 352 33614 9	
☐ IN PURSUIT OF ANNA Natasha Rostova	ISBN 978 0 352 34060 3	
☐ IN THE FLESH Emma Holly	ISBN 978 0 352 34117 4	
☐ LEARNING TO LOVE IT Alison Tyler	ISBN 978 0 352 33535 7	
☐ MAD ABOUT THE BOY Mathilde Madden	ISBN 978 0 352 34001 6	
☐ MAKE YOU A MAN Anna Clare	ISBN 978 0 352 34006 1	
☐ MAN HUNT Cathleen Ross	ISBN 978 0 352 33583 8	
☐ THE MASTER OF SHILDEN Lucinda Carrington	ISBN 978 0 352 33140 3	
☐ MIXED DOUBLES Zoe le Verdier	ISBN 978 0 352 33312 4	£6.99
☐ MIXED SIGNALS Anna Clare	ISBN 978 0 352 33889 1	£6.99
☐ MS BEHAVIOUR Mini Lee	ISBN 978 0 352 33962 1	
☐ PACKING HEAT Karina Moore	ISBN 978 0 352 33356 8	£6.99
☐ PAGAN HEAT Monica Belle	ISBN 978 0 352 33974 4	

☐ PEEP SHOW Mathilde Madden   ISBN 978 0 352 33924 9

☐ THE PRIVATE UNDOING OF A PUBLIC SERVANT   ISBN 978 0 352 34066 5
    Leonie Martel

☐ RUDE AWAKENING Pamela Kyle   ISBN 978 0 352 33036 9

☐ SAUCE FOR THE GOOSE Mary Rose Maxwell   ISBN 978 0 352 33492 3

☐ SPLIT Kristina Lloyd   ISBN 978 0 352 34154 9

☐ STELLA DOES HOLLYWOOD Stella Black   ISBN 978 0 352 33588 3

☐ THE STRANGER Portia Da Costa   ISBN 978 0 352 33211 0

☐ SUITE SEVENTEEN Portia Da Costa   ISBN 978 0 352 34109 9

☐ TONGUE IN CHEEK Tabitha Flyte   ISBN 978 0 352 33484 8

☐ THE TOP OF HER GAME Emma Holly   ISBN 978 0 352 34116 7

☐ UNNATURAL SELECTION Alaine Hood   ISBN 978 0 352 33963 8

☐ VELVET GLOVE Emma Holly   ISBN 978 0 352 34115 0

☐ VILLAGE OF SECRETS Mercedes Kelly   ISBN 978 0 352 33344 5

☐ WILD BY NATURE Monica Belle   ISBN 978 0 352 33915 7   £6.99

☐ WING OF MADNESS Mae Nixon   ISBN 978 0 352 34099 3

BLACK LACE BOOKS WITH AN HISTORICAL SETTING

☐ THE BARBARIAN GEISHA Charlotte Royal   ISBN 978 0 352 33267 7

☐ BARBARIAN PRIZE Deanna Ashford   ISBN 978 0 352 34017 7

☐ THE CAPTIVATION Natasha Rostova   ISBN 978 0 352 33234 9

☐ DARKER THAN LOVE Kristina Lloyd   ISBN 978 0 352 33279 0

☐ WILD KINGDOM Deanna Ashford   ISBN 978 0 352 33549 4

☐ DIVINE TORMENT Janine Ashbless   ISBN 978 0 352 33719 1

☐ FRENCH MANNERS Olivia Christie   ISBN 978 0 352 33214 1

☐ LORD WRAXALL'S FANCY Anna Lieff Saxby   ISBN 978 0 352 33080 2

☐ NICOLE'S REVENGE Lisette Allen   ISBN 978 0 352 32984 4

☐ THE SENSES BEJEWELLED Cleo Cordell   ISBN 978 0 352 32904 2   £6.99

☐ THE SOCIETY OF SIN Sian Lacey Taylder   ISBN 978 0 352 34080 1

☐ TEMPLAR PRIZE Deanna Ashford   ISBN 978 0 352 34137 2

☐ UNDRESSING THE DEVIL Angel Strand   ISBN 978 0 352 33938 6

BLACK LACE BOOKS WITH A PARANORMAL THEME

☐ BRIGHT FIRE Maya Hess   ISBN 978 0 352 34104 4

☐ BURNING BRIGHT Janine Ashbless   ISBN 978 0 352 34085 6

☐ CRUEL ENCHANTMENT Janine Ashbless   ISBN 978 0 352 33483 1

❑ FLOOD Anna Clare ISBN 978 0 352 34094 8
❑ GOTHIC BLUE Portia Da Costa ISBN 978 0 352 33075 8
❑ THE PRIDE Edie Bingham ISBN 978 0 352 33997 3
❑ THE SILVER COLLAR Mathilde Madden ISBN 978 0 352 34141 9
❑ THE TEN VISIONS Olivia Knight ISBN 978 0 352 34119 8

BLACK LACE ANTHOLOGIES

❑ BLACK LACE QUICKIES 1 Various ISBN 978 0 352 34126 6 £2.99
❑ BLACK LACE QUICKIES 2 Various ISBN 978 0 352 34127 3 £2.99
❑ BLACK LACE QUICKIES 3 Various ISBN 978 0 352 34128 0 £2.99
❑ BLACK LACE QUICKIES 4 Various ISBN 978 0 352 34129 7 £2.99
❑ BLACK LACE QUICKIES 5 Various ISBN 978 0 352 34130 3 £2.99
❑ BLACK LACE QUICKIES 6 Various ISBN 978 0 352 34133 4 £2.99
❑ BLACK LACE QUICKIES 7 Various ISBN 978 0 352 34146 4 £2.99
❑ BLACK LACE QUICKIES 8 Various ISBN 978 0 352 34147 1 £2.99
❑ BLACK LACE QUICKIES 9 Various ISBN 978 0 352 34155 6 £2.99
❑ MORE WICKED WORDS Various ISBN 978 0 352 33487 9 £6.99
❑ WICKED WORDS 3 Various ISBN 978 0 352 33522 7 £6.99
❑ WICKED WORDS 4 Various ISBN 978 0 352 33603 3 £6.99
❑ WICKED WORDS 5 Various ISBN 978 0 352 33642 2 £6.99
❑ WICKED WORDS 6 Various ISBN 978 0 352 33690 3 £6.99
❑ WICKED WORDS 7 Various ISBN 978 0 352 33743 6 £6.99
❑ WICKED WORDS 8 Various ISBN 978 0 352 33787 0 £6.99
❑ WICKED WORDS 9 Various ISBN 978 0 352 33860 0
❑ WICKED WORDS 10 Various ISBN 978 0 352 33893 8
❑ THE BEST OF BLACK LACE 2 Various ISBN 978 0 352 33718 4
❑ WICKED WORDS: SEX IN THE OFFICE Various ISBN 978 0 352 33944 7
❑ WICKED WORDS: SEX AT THE SPORTS CLUB Various ISBN 978 0 352 33991 1
❑ WICKED WORDS: SEX ON HOLIDAY Various ISBN 978 0 352 33961 4
❑ WICKED WORDS: SEX IN UNIFORM Various ISBN 978 0 352 34002 3
❑ WICKED WORDS: SEX IN THE KITCHEN Various ISBN 978 0 352 34018 4
❑ WICKED WORDS: SEX ON THE MOVE Various ISBN 978 0 352 34034 4
❑ WICKED WORDS: SEX AND MUSIC Various ISBN 978 0 352 34061 0
❑ WICKED WORDS: SEX AND SHOPPING Various ISBN 978 0 352 34076 4
❑ SEX IN PUBLIC Various ISBN 978 0 352 34089 4
❑ SEX WITH STRANGERS Various ISBN 978 0 352 34105 1

To find out the latest information about Black Lace titles, check out the website: www.black-lace-books.com or send for a booklist with complete synopses by writing to:

Black Lace Booklist, Virgin Books Ltd
Thames Wharf Studios
Rainville Road
London W6 9HA

Please include an SAE of decent size. Please note only British stamps are valid.

Our privacy policy
We will not disclose information you supply us to any other parties. We will not disclose any information which identifies you personally to any person without your express consent.

From time to time we may send out information about Black Lace books and special offers. Please tick here if you do <u>not</u> wish to receive Black Lace information. ❏

Please send me the books I have ticked above.

Name...

Address...

....

....

....

Post Code..

Send to: Virgin Books Cash Sales, Thames Wharf Studios, Rainville Road, London W6 9HA.

US customers: for prices and details of how to order books for delivery by mail, call 888-330-8477.

Please enclose a cheque or postal order, made payable to Virgin Books Ltd, to the value of the books you have ordered plus postage and packing costs as follows:

UK and BFPO – £1.00 for the first book, 50p for each subsequent book.

Overseas (including Republic of Ireland) – £2.00 for the first book, £1.00 for each subsequent book.

If you would prefer to pay by VISA, ACCESS/MASTERCARD, DINERS CLUB, AMEX or SWITCH, please write your card number and expiry date here:..

....

Signature...

Please allow up to 28 days for delivery.